BASIC AND CLINICAL SCIENCE COURSE

Lens and Cataract

Section 11

2007–2008

(Last major revision 2004–2005)

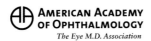

AMERICAN ACADEMY OF OPHTHALMOLOGY
The Eye M.D. Association

LEO

LIFELONG
EDUCATION FOR THE
OPHTHALMOLOGIST®

The Basic and Clinical Science Course is one component of the Lifelong Education for the Ophthalmologist (LEO) framework, which assists members in planning their continuing medical education. LEO includes an array of clinical education products that members may select to form individualized, self-directed learning plans for updating their clinical knowledge. Active members or fellows who use LEO components may accumulate sufficient CME credits to earn the LEO Award. Contact the Academy's Clinical Education Division for further information on LEO.

The Academy provides this material for educational purposes only. It is not intended to represent the only or best method or procedure in every case, nor to replace a physician's own judgment or give specific advice for case management. Including all indications, contraindications, side effects, and alternative agents for each drug or treatment is beyond the scope of this material. All information and recommendations should be verified, prior to use, with current information included in the manufacturers' package inserts or other independent sources, and considered in light of the patient's condition and history. Reference to certain drugs, instruments, and other products in this publication is made for illustrative purposes only and is not intended to constitute an endorsement of such. Some material may include information on applications that are not considered community standard, that reflect indications not included in approved FDA labeling, or that are approved for use only in restricted research settings. The FDA has stated that it is the responsibility of the physician to determine the FDA status of each drug or device he or she wishes to use, and to use them with appropriate patient consent in compliance with applicable law. The Academy specifically disclaims any and all liability for injury or other damages of any kind, from negligence or otherwise, for any and all claims that may arise from the use of, any recommendations or other information contained herein.

Basic and Clinical Science Course

Thomas J. Liesegang, MD, Jacksonville, Florida, *Senior Secretary for Clinical Education*

Gregory L. Skuta, MD, Oklahoma City, Oklahoma, *Secretary for Ophthalmic Knowledge*

Louis B. Cantor, MD, Indianapolis, Indiana, *BCSC Course Chair*

Section 11

Faculty Responsible for This Edition

Steven I. Rosenfeld, MD, *Chair*, Delray Beach, Florida
Mark H. Blecher, MD, Philadelphia, Pennsylvania
James C. Bobrow, MD, Clayton, Missouri
Cynthia A. Bradford, MD, Oklahoma City, Oklahoma
David Glasser, MD, Columbia, Maryland
John S. Berestka, MD, Wayzata, Minnesota
    Practicing Ophthalmologists Advisory Committee for Education

The authors state the following financial relationships:
Dr. Rosenfeld: Speakers' Bureau, Allergan

The other authors state that they have no significant financial interest or other relationship with the manufacturer of any commercial product discussed in the chapters that they contributed to this publication or with the manufacturer of any competing commercial product.

Recent Past Faculty

L. Michael Cobo, MD	Mariannette J. Miller-Meeks, MD
Robert S. Feder, MD	Priscilla E. Perry, MD
Lawrence A. Gans, MD	Thomas J. Roussel, MD
M. Bowes Hamill, MD	David J. Schanzlin, MD
Karla J. Johns, MD	Woodford S. Van Meter, MD

In addition, the Academy gratefully acknowledges the contributions of numerous past faculty and advisory committee members who have played an important role in the development of previous editions of the Basic and Clinical Science Course.

American Academy of Ophthalmology Staff

Richard A. Zorab, *Vice President, Ophthalmic Knowledge*
Hal Straus, *Director, Publications Department*
Carol L. Dondrea, *Publications Manager*
Christine Arturo, *Acquisitions Manager*
Nicole DuCharme, *Production Manager*
Stephanie Tanaka, *Medical Editor*
Steven Huebner, *Administrative Coordinator*

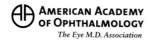

**AMERICAN ACADEMY
OF OPHTHALMOLOGY**
The Eye M.D. Association

655 Beach Street
Box 7424
San Francisco, CA 94120-7424

Contents

8   Surgery for Cataract   89

General Introduction

The Basic and Clinical Science Course (BCSC) is designed to meet the needs of residents and practitioners for a comprehensive yet concise curriculum of the field of ophthalmology. The BCSC has developed from its original brief outline format, which relied heavily on outside readings, to a more convenient and educationally useful self-contained text. The Academy updates and revises the course annually, with the goals of integrating the basic science and clinical practice of ophthalmology and of keeping ophthalmologists current with new developments in the various subspecialties.

The BCSC incorporates the effort and expertise of more than 80 ophthalmologists, organized into 13 section faculties, working with Academy editorial staff. In addition, the course continues to benefit from many lasting contributions made by the faculties of previous editions. Members of the Academy's Practicing Ophthalmologists Advisory Committee for Education serve on each faculty and, as a group, review every volume before and after major revisions.

Organization of the Course

The Basic and Clinical Science Course comprises 13 volumes, incorporating fundamental ophthalmic knowledge, subspecialty areas, and special topics:

1. Update on General Medicine
2. Fundamentals and Principles of Ophthalmology
3. Clinical Optics
4. Ophthalmic Pathology and Intraocular Tumors
5. Neuro-Ophthalmology
6. Pediatric Ophthalmology and Strabismus
7. Orbit, Eyelids, and Lacrimal System
8. External Disease and Cornea
9. Intraocular Inflammation and Uveitis
10. Glaucoma
11. Lens and Cataract
12. Retina and Vitreous
13. Refractive Surgery

In addition, a comprehensive Master Index allows the reader to easily locate subjects throughout the entire series.

References

Readers who wish to explore specific topics in greater detail may consult the journal references cited within each chapter and the Basic Texts listed at the back of the book.

These references are intended to be selective rather than exhaustive, chosen by the BCSC faculty as being important, current, and readily available to residents and practitioners.

Related Academy educational materials are also listed in the appropriate sections. They include books, audiovisual materials, self-assessment programs, clinical modules, and interactive programs.

Study Questions and CME Credit

Each volume of the BCSC is designed as an independent study activity for ophthalmology residents and practitioners. The learning objectives for this volume are given on page 1. The text, illustrations, and references provide the information necessary to achieve the objectives; the study questions allow readers to test their understanding of the material and their mastery of the objectives. Physicians who wish to claim CME credit for this educational activity may do so by mail, fax, or online. The necessary forms and instructions are given at the end of the book.

Conclusion

The Basic and Clinical Science Course has expanded greatly over the years, with the addition of much new text and numerous illustrations. Recent editions have sought to place a greater emphasis on clinical applicability, while maintaining a solid foundation in basic science. As with any educational program, it reflects the experience of its authors. As its faculties change and as medicine progresses, new viewpoints are always emerging on controversial subjects and techniques. Not all alternate approaches can be included in this series; as with any educational endeavor, the learner should seek additional sources, including such carefully balanced opinions as the Academy's Preferred Practice Patterns.

The BCSC faculty and staff are continuously striving to improve the educational usefulness of the course; you, the reader, can contribute to this ongoing process. If you have any suggestions or questions about the series, please do not hesitate to contact the faculty or the editors.

The authors, editors, and reviewers hope that your study of the BCSC will be of lasting value and that each section will serve as a practical resource for quality patient care.

Objectives

Upon completion of BCSC Section 11, *Lens and Cataract*, the reader should be able to:

- Describe the normal anatomy, embryologic development, physiology, and biochemistry of the crystalline lens

- Identify congenital anomalies of the lens

- Distinguish types of congenital and acquired cataracts

- Describe the association of cataracts with aging, trauma, medications, and systemic and ocular diseases

- Appropriately evaluate and manage patients with cataract and other lens abnormalities

- Explain the principles of cataract surgery techniques and associated surgical technology

- Develop an appropriate differential diagnosis and management plan for intra-operative and postoperative complications of cataract surgery

- Identify special circumstances in which cataract surgery techniques should be modified and develop appropriate treatment plans

Introduction

The ancient Greeks and Romans believed that the lens was the part of the eye responsible for the faculty of seeing. They theorized that the optic nerves were hollow channels through which "visual spirits" traveled from the brain to meet visual rays from the outside world at the lens, which they thought was located in the center of the globe. The visual information would then flow back to the brain. This concept was known as the *emanation theory of vision.* Celsus (25 BC–AD 50) drew the lens in the center of the globe, with an empty space called the *locus vacuus* anterior to it, in AD 30 (Fig I-1).

These erroneous ideas about lens position and function persisted through the Middle Ages and into the Renaissance, as shown by the drawings of the Belgian anatomist Andreas Vesalius in 1543 (Fig I-2). However, the true position of the crystalline lens was illustrated by the Italian anatomist Fabricius ab Aquapendente in 1600 (Fig I-3); and the Swiss physician Felix Plater (1536–1614) first postulated that the retina, and not the lens, was the part of the eye responsible for sight.

Today, many areas of lens physiology and biochemistry are still subjects of active research. No medical treatment, for example, can yet prevent the formation or progression of cataract in the lens of the otherwise healthy adult eye, and theories about cataract formation and innovative forms of management continue to be controversial. Although various risk factors for cataract development (ultraviolet B radiation, diabetes, drug use,

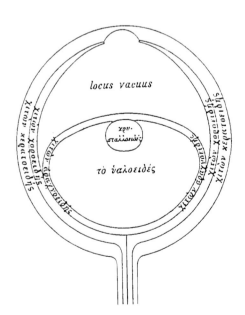

Figure I-1 The eye, after Celsus. *(From Gorin G.* History of Ophthalmology. *Wilmington: Publish or Perish, Inc; 1982.)*

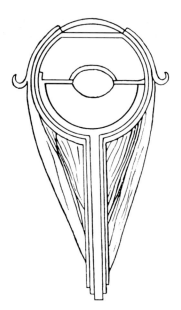

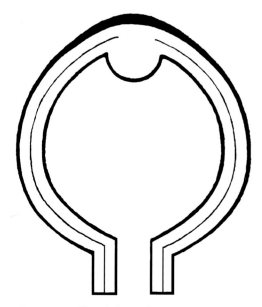

Figure I-2 Schematic eye from *De fabrica corporis humani* of Andreas Vesalius (1514–1564). *(Reproduced by permission from the Ophthalmic Publishing Company. Feigenbaum A. Early history of cataract and the ancient operation for cataract. Am J Ophthalmol. 1960;49:307.)*

Figure I-3 Sketch from *De oculo* of Fabricius ab Aquapendente (1537–1619), showing correct position of the lens within the eyeball. *(Reproduced by permission from the Ophthalmic Publishing Company. Feigenbaum A. Early history of cataract and the ancient operation for cataract. Am J Ophthalmol. 1960;49:307.)*

smoking, diarrhea, alcohol use, and oxidative damage) have been identified, data to develop guidelines for reducing the risk of cataract remain insufficient.

Cataract is the leading cause of preventable blindness in the world, whereas cataract extraction with intraocular lens (IOL) implantation is perhaps the most effective surgical procedure in all of medicine. More than 1.3 million cataract procedures are performed in the United States each year, and the visual disability associated with cataract formation accounts for over 8 million physician office visits each year.

The prevalence of lens disorders and continuing developments in their management make the basic and clinical science of the lens an important subject in ophthalmology training. The goal of Section 11 is to provide a curriculum for the study of all aspects of the lens, including the structure and function of the normal lens, the features of diseases involving the lens, and the surgical management of lens abnormalities, such as recent developments in phacoemulsification and laser capsulotomy. Because the specifics of surgical techniques and instrumentation are continuously changing, the authors of this volume have chosen to provide a balanced presentation of the general principles of cataract management, emphasizing the major prevailing approaches.

In addition, to help put today's techniques into perspective, historical vignettes describing the evolution of cataract surgery and IOL implantation appear at the beginning of Chapter 8 and in the discussion of IOLs later in that chapter.

CHAPTER 1

Anatomy

Normal Crystalline Lens

The crystalline lens is a transparent, biconvex structure whose functions are

- to maintain its own clarity
- to refract light
- to provide accommodation

The lens has no blood supply or innervation after fetal development, and it depends entirely on the aqueous humor to meet its metabolic requirements and to carry off its wastes. It lies posterior to the iris and anterior to the vitreous body (Fig 1-1). It is suspended in position by the zonules of Zinn, consisting of delicate yet strong fibers that support and attach it to the ciliary body. The lens is composed of the capsule, lens epithelium, cortex, and nucleus (Fig 1-2).

The anterior and posterior poles of the lens are joined by an imaginary line called the *axis*, which passes through them. Lines on the surface passing from one pole to the other are referred to as *meridians*. The *equator* of the lens is its greatest circumference.

The lens is able to refract light because its index of refraction—normally about 1.4 centrally and 1.36 peripherally—is different from that of the aqueous and vitreous that surround it. In its nonaccommodative state, the lens contributes about 15–20 diopters (D) of the approximately 60 D of convergent refractive power of the average human eye. The remaining 40 or so diopters of convergent refractive power occur at the air–cornea interface.

The lens continues to grow throughout life. At birth, it measures approximately 6.4 mm equatorially and 3.5 mm anteroposteriorly and weighs about 90 mg. The adult lens typically measures 9 mm equatorially and 5 mm anteroposteriorly and weighs approximately 255 mg. The relative thickness of the cortex increases with age. At the same time, the lens adopts an increasingly curved shape so that older lenses have more refractive power. However, the index of refraction decreases with age, probably as a result of the increasing presence of insoluble protein particles. Thus, the aging eye may become either more hyperopic or myopic with age, depending on the balance of these opposing changes.

Capsule

The lens capsule is an elastic, transparent basement membrane composed of type IV collagen laid down by the epithelial cells. The capsule contains the lens substance and is capable of molding it during accommodative changes. The outer layer of the lens capsule,

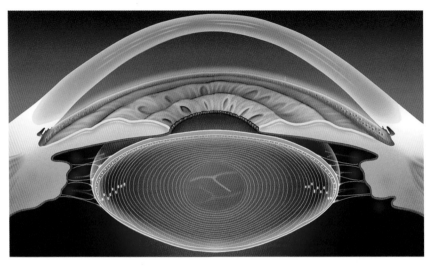

Figure 1-1 Cross section of the human crystalline lens, showing its relationship to surrounding ocular structures. *(Illustration by Christine Gralapp.)*

the *zonular lamella,* also serves as the point of attachment for the zonular fibers. The lens capsule is thickest in the anterior and posterior preequatorial zones and thinnest in the region of the central posterior pole, where it may be as thin as 2–4 μm. The anterior lens capsule is considerably thicker than the posterior capsule at birth and increases in thickness throughout life (Fig 1-3).

Zonular Fibers

The lens is supported by zonular fibers that originate from basal laminae of the nonpigmented epithelium of the pars plana and pars plicata of the ciliary body. These zonular fibers insert on the lens capsule in the equatorial region in a continuous fashion, anteriorly 1.5 mm onto the anterior lens capsule and posteriorly 1.25 mm onto the posterior lens capsule. With age, the equatorial zonular fibers regress, leaving separate anterior and posterior layers that appear in a triangular shape on cross section of the zonular ring. The fibers are 5–30 μm in diameter; light microscopy shows them to be eosinophilic structures that have a positive periodic acid–Schiff (PAS) reaction. Ultrastructurally, the fibers are composed of strands, or fibrils, 8–10 nm in diameter with 12–14 nm of banding.

Lens Epithelium

Immediately behind the anterior lens capsule is a single layer of epithelial cells. These cells are metabolically active and carry out all normal cell activities, including the biosynthesis of DNA, RNA, protein, and lipid; they also generate ATP to meet the energy demands of the lens. The epithelial cells are mitotic, with the greatest activity of premitotic (replicative, or S-phase) DNA synthesis occurring in a ring around the anterior lens known as the *germinative zone.* These newly formed cells migrate toward the equator,

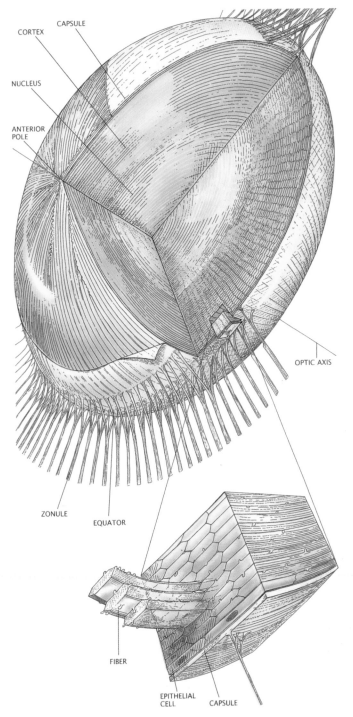

CORTEX

CAPSULE

NUCLEUS

ANTERIOR
POLE

OPTIC AXIS

ZONULE

EQUATOR

FIBER

EPITHELIAL
CELL

CAPSULE

Figure 1-2 Structure of the normal human lens. *(Illustration by Carol Donner. Reproduced with permission from Koretz JF, Handelman GH. How the human eye focuses.* Scientific American. *July 1988:94.)*

where they differentiate into fibers. As the epithelial cells migrate toward the bow region of the lens, they begin the process of terminal differentiation into lens fibers (Fig 1-4).

Perhaps the most dramatic morphologic change occurs when the epithelial cells elongate to form lens fiber cells. This change is associated with a tremendous increase in the mass of cellular proteins in the membranes of each individual fiber cell. At the same time, the cells lose organelles, including cell nuclei, mitochondria, and ribosomes. The loss of these organelles is optically advantageous because light passing through the lens is no longer absorbed or scattered by these structures. However, because these new lens

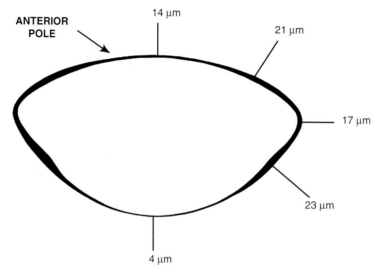

Figure 1-3 Schematic of adult human lens capsule showing relative thickness of capsule in different zones. *(Illustration by Christine Gralapp.)*

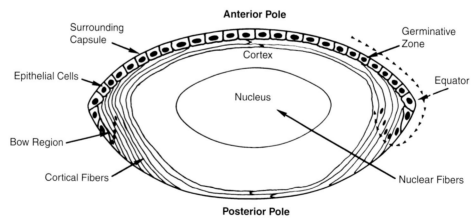

Figure 1-4 Schematic of the mammalian lens in cross section. Arrowheads indicate direction of cell migration from the epithelium to the cortex. *(From Anderson RE, ed. Biochemistry of the Eye. San Francisco: American Academy of Ophthalmology; 1983;6:112.)*

fiber cells lack the metabolic functions previously carried out by the organelles, they are now dependent on glycolysis for energy production (see Chapter 2).

Nucleus and Cortex

No cells are lost from the lens; as new fibers are laid down, they crowd and compact the previously formed fibers, with the oldest layers being the most central. The oldest of these, the *embryonic* and *fetal lens nuclei*, were produced in embryonic life and persist in the center of the lens (see Fig 4-1 in Chapter 4). The outermost fibers are the most recently formed and make up the cortex of the lens.

Lens sutures are formed by the arrangement of interdigitations of apical cell processes *(anterior sutures)* and basal cell processes *(posterior sutures)*. In addition to the Y-sutures located within the lens nucleus, multiple optical zones are visible by slit-lamp biomicroscopy. These zones of demarcation occur because strata of epithelial cells with differing optical densities are laid down throughout life. There is no distinct morphologic differentiation between the cortex and nucleus; rather, the transition between these regions is gradual. Although some surgical texts make distinctions among the nucleus, epinucleus, and cortex, these terms relate only to potential differences in the behavior and appearance of the material during surgical procedures.

Kuszak JR, Clark JI, Cooper KE, et al. Biology of the lens: lens transparency as a function of embryology, anatomy and physiology. In: Albert DM, Jakobiec FA, eds. *Principles and Practice of Ophthalmology*. 2nd ed. Philadelphia: Saunders; 2000:1355–1408.

Snell RS, Lemp MA. *Clinical Anatomy of the Eye*. 2nd ed. Boston: Blackwell; 1998:197–204.

CHAPTER 2

Biochemistry

Molecular Biology

Crystallin Proteins

The human lens has a protein concentration of 33% of its wet weight, which is twice that of most other tissues. Lens proteins can be divided into 2 groups based on their water solubility (Fig 2-1). The water-soluble fraction accounts for about 80% of lens proteins and consists mainly of a group of proteins called *crystallins*. The crystallins are intracellular proteins contained within the epithelium and plasma membrane of the lens fiber cells. They have traditionally been subdivided into 3 major groups: alpha, beta, and gamma. However, accumulated evidence, including DNA sequencing, indicates that the beta and gamma crystallins are part of the same family; and they are now generally referred to as the *betagamma crystallins*.

Alpha crystallins represent 32% of the lens proteins. They are the largest, with a molecular weight ranging from 600 to 4000 kiloDaltons (kD), depending on the tendency of subunits to aggregate. The alpha crystallins are not one discrete protein but are composed of a mixture of different-sized macromolecular aggregates of 4 major subunits and up to 9 minor subunits. Each subunit polypeptide has a molecular weight of about 20 kD,

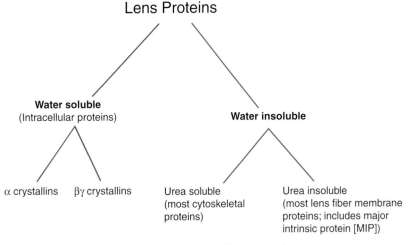

Figure 2-1 Overview of lens proteins.

and the chains are held together by hydrogen bonds and hydrophobic interactions. Alpha crystallins appear to be specifically involved with the transformation of epithelial cells into lens fibers. The rate of synthesis of alpha crystallins is 7 times higher in epithelial cells than in the cortical fibers, indicating a significant decrease in rate of synthesis after the transformation.

Beta and gamma crystallins have historically been discussed separately because certain basic properties such as their isoelectric points and aggregation properties differ. However, the two crystallins have homologous amino acid sequences and similar structures and share an evolutionary history, so they can be thought of as part of a family of proteins. By gel chromatography, the family can be separated into beta H, beta L, and gamma crystallins. The *beta crystallins* account for 55% (by weight) of the water-soluble proteins in the lens. Three fractions of different molecular weight have been identified; they appear to be composed of largely identical subunits that are very closely related immunochemically. The basic structure of these crystallins has been maintained through hundreds of millions of years of vertebrate evolution.

The *gamma crystallins* are the smallest of the crystallins, with a molecular weight in the range of 20 kD. They make up approximately 1.5% of adult mammal lens protein but constitute as much as 60% of soluble lens protein in weanling animals. X-ray crystallographic studies have determined the 3-dimensional structure of the gamma crystallins to high resolution. Fourfold repetition in the 3-dimensional structure suggests that gamma crystallins might have arisen from double duplication and fusion of a gene for a 40-residue polypeptide.

Membrane Structural Proteins and Cytoskeletal Proteins

The water-insoluble fraction of lens proteins can be further separated into two fractions, one soluble and one insoluble in 8 molar urea. The *urea-soluble fraction* contains cytoskeletal proteins that provide the structural framework of the lens cells. The *urea-insoluble fraction* contains the lens fiber plasma membranes that resemble erythrocyte plasma membranes in many respects. Several proteins are associated with these fiber plasma membranes. One makes up nearly 50% of the membrane proteins and has come to be known as the *major intrinsic protein (MIP)*. This protein, with a molecular weight of 28 kD, breaks down with age to a 22-kD protein. The relative proportions of these two proteins become about equal at 20–30 years of age. The 22-kD protein predominates in the nucleus. The MIP first appears in the lens just as the fibers begin to elongate and can be detected in membranes throughout the mass of the lens. It is not found in the epithelial cells at all, however, and thus seems to be associated with the differentiation of epithelial cells into fiber cells. The MIP, concentrated in the gap junctions, is the predominant protein of the junction-enriched membrane proteins. It is an inherent part of the membrane, where it has been localized by immunofluorescence.

Increase of Water-Insoluble Proteins With Age

Regarding water solubility, one hypothesis suggests that, over time, lens proteins become water insoluble and aggregate to form very large particles that scatter light, thus producing lens opacities. Some researchers have attempted to correlate higher percentages of water-insoluble proteins with increased lens opacification, but this hypothesis remains controversial. It should be noted that the water-insoluble protein fraction increases with age even if the lens remains clear. Conversion of the water-soluble proteins into water-insoluble proteins appears to be a natural process in lens fiber maturation, but it may be accelerated or occur to excess in certain cataractous lenses.

In cataracts with significant browning of the lens nucleus *(brunescent cataracts),* the increase in the amount of water-insoluble protein does correlate with the degree of opacification. In markedly brunescent cataracts, as much as 90% of the nuclear proteins are insoluble. Associated oxidative changes occur, including protein-to-protein and protein-to-glutathione disulfide bond formation, decreased reduced glutathione, and increased glutathione disulfide. Membrane-associated methionine and cysteine also become oxidized.

In the young lens, most of the water-insoluble proteins can be dissolved in urea. With age and, more notably, with brunescent nuclear cataract formation, the nuclear proteins become increasingly insoluble in urea. In addition to the increases in disulfide linkages, these nuclear proteins are highly cross-linked by nondisulfide bonds. This insoluble protein fraction contains a yellow-to-brown protein that is found in high concentration in nuclear cataracts. Increased fluorescence in the lens (not produced from tryptophan) is associated with the nondisulfide cross-links that form in brunescent nuclear cataracts.

Decrease in Lens Protein Concentration With Age

Although aging brings about a natural decrease in the absolute amount of protein in the lens, this reduction is even more remarkable in cataractous lenses. As mentioned earlier, the percentage of soluble proteins also decreases, from approximately 81% in adult transparent lenses to only 51.4% in cataractous lenses. Loss of proteins from the lens probably represents an escape of intact crystallins through the lens capsule. Researchers have found that, in cortical cataracts, the levels of both alpha and gamma crystallins in the aqueous humor increase; in nuclear cataracts, the level of alpha crystallins increases, whereas that of gamma crystallins decreases.

Evolution and the Molecular Biology of Crystallins

Research in DNA sequencing has led to the interesting discovery that alpha crystallins are closely related to proteins found in diverse animals and sites, such as a heat-shock protein in the fruit fly *Drosophila* and an egg antigen in the blood fluke *Schistosoma mansoni.* It is theorized that the common gene sequence produces a highly stable structural unit that helps protect the protein from degradation in a stressful environment. This successful and stable gene product is seen in many diverse situations in nature.

Hejtmancik JF, Piatigorsky J. Lens proteins and their molecular biology. In: Albert DM, Jakobiec FA, eds. *Principles and Practice of Ophthalmology.* 2nd ed. Philadelphia: Saunders; 2000:1409–1428.

Carbohydrate Metabolism

The goal of lens metabolism is the maintenance of transparency. In the lens, energy production largely depends on glucose metabolism. Glucose enters the lens from the aqueous both by *simple diffusion* and by a mediated transfer process called *facilitated diffusion*. Most of the glucose transported into the lens is phosphorylated to a glucose-6-phosphate (G6P) by the enzyme hexokinase. This reaction is 70–1000 times slower than that of other enzymes involved in lens glycolysis and is, therefore, rate limited in the lens. Once formed, G6P enters one of two metabolic pathways: anaerobic glycolysis or the hexose monophosphate (HMP) shunt (Fig 2-2).

The more active of these two pathways is anaerobic glycolysis, which provides most of the high-energy phosphate bonds required for lens metabolism. Substrate-linked phosphorylation of ADP to ATP occurs at two steps along the way to lactate. The rate-limiting step in the glycolytic pathway itself is at the level of the enzyme phosphofructokinase, which is regulated through feedback control by metabolic products of the glycolytic pathway. This pathway is much less efficient than aerobic glycolysis because only 2 net molecules of ATP are produced for each glucose molecule utilized, whereas aerobic glycolysis produces an additional 36 molecules of ATP from each glucose molecule metabolized in the citric acid cycle (oxidative metabolism). Because of the low oxygen tension in the lens, only about 3% of the lens glucose passes through the Krebs citric acid cycle to produce ATP; however, even this low level of aerobic metabolism produces about 25% of the lens ATP.

That the lens is not dependent on oxygen is demonstrated by its ability to sustain normal metabolism in a nitrogen environment. Provided with ample glucose, the anoxic in vitro lens remains completely transparent, has normal levels of ATP, and maintains its ion and amino acid pump activities. However, when deprived of glucose, the lens cannot maintain these functions and becomes hazy after several hours, even in the presence of oxygen.

The less active pathway for utilization of G6P in the lens is the hexose monophosphate (HMP) shunt, also known as the pentose phosphate pathway. About 5% of lens glucose is metabolized by this route, although the pathway is stimulated in the presence of elevated levels of glucose. The activity of the HMP shunt is higher in the lens than in most tissues, but its role is far from established. As in other tissues, it may provide NADPH (the reduced form of nicotinamide-adenine dinucleotide phosphate [NADP]) for fatty acid biosynthesis and ribose for nucleotide biosynthesis. It also provides the NADPH necessary for glutathione reductase and aldose reductase activities in the lens. The carbohydrate products of the HMP shunt enter the glycolytic pathway and are metabolized to lactate.

Aldose reductase is the key enzyme in yet another pathway for lens sugar metabolism, the *sorbitol pathway*. This enzyme has been found to play a pivotal role in the development of "sugar" cataracts. [See also the biochemistry chapters (Part IV) in BCSC Section 2, *Fundamentals and Principles of Ophthalmology,* especially Chapter 14.] The Michaelis-Menten equation explains the reaction velocity, V, as a function of the enzyme and substrate concentrations and the Michaelis constant, K_m. Also known as the affinity

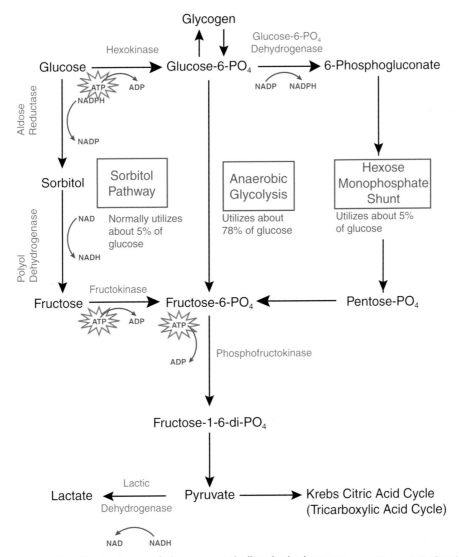

Figure 2-2 Simplified scheme of glucose metabolism in the lens. *(Adapted with permission from Hart WM Jr, ed. Adler's Physiology of the Eye: Clinical Application. 9th ed. St Louis: Mosby; 1992:362.)*

constant, K_m is equal to the substrate concentration at which the reaction rate is half of its maximal value. A high K_m indicates weak binding; a low K_m indicates strong binding. The affinity constant K_m for aldose reductase is about 700 times that for hexokinase. Because the affinity is actually the inverse of K_m, aldose reductase has a very low affinity for glucose compared to hexokinase. Less than 4% of lens glucose is normally converted to sorbitol.

As previously noted, the hexokinase reaction is rate-limited in phosphorylating glucose in the lens and is inhibited by the feedback mechanisms of the products of glycolysis. Therefore, when glucose increases in the lens, as occurs in hyperglycemic states, the sorbitol pathway is activated relatively more than glycolysis, and sorbitol accumulates. Sorbitol is metabolized to fructose by the enzyme polyol dehydrogenase. Unfortunately, this enzyme has a relatively low affinity (high K_m), meaning that considerable sorbitol will accumulate before being further metabolized. This characteristic, combined with the poor permeability of the lens to sorbitol, results in retention of sorbitol in the lens.

A high NADPH/NADH ratio drives the reaction in the forward direction. The accumulation of NADP that occurs as a consequence of activation of the sorbitol pathway may cause the stimulation of the HMP shunt that is observed in the presence of elevated lens glucose. Along with sorbitol, fructose also builds up in a lens incubated in a high-glucose environment. Together, the two sugars increase the osmotic pressure within the lens, drawing in water. At first, the energy-dependent pumps of the lens are able to compensate, but ultimately they are overwhelmed. The result is swelling of the fibers, disruption of the normal cytoskeletal architecture, and lens opacification.

Galactose is also a substrate for aldose reductase, producing the alcohol galactitol (dulcitol). Galactitol, however, is not a substrate for sugar alcohol dehydrogenase and thus accumulates rapidly, producing the same osmotic effects—and the same consequences—as sorbitol. Excess production of galactitol occurs in patients with inborn disorders of galactose metabolism.

The patient with an inborn error of galactose metabolism is unable to utilize galactose properly and accumulates galactitol and other galactose metabolites. Galactose cataracts can be induced experimentally in animals by maintaining them on diets extremely rich in galactose.

The pivotal role of aldose reductase in cataractogenesis in animals is apparent from studies of the development of sugar-induced cataract in various animal species. Those species that have high aldose reductase activities develop lens opacities, whereas those lacking aldose reductase do not. In addition, specific inhibitors of this enzymatic activity, applied either systemically or topically to one eye, decrease the rate of onset and severity of sugar cataracts in experimental studies.

Oxidative Damage and Protective Mechanisms

Free radicals are generated in the course of normal cellular metabolic activities and may also be produced by external agents such as radiant energy. These highly reactive free radicals can lead to the damage of lens fibers. Peroxidation of fiber plasma or lens fiber plasma membrane lipids has been suggested as a factor contributing to lens opacification. In the process of lipid peroxidation, the oxidizing agent removes a hydrogen atom from the polyunsaturated fatty acid, forming a fatty acid radical, which, in turn, attacks molecular oxygen, forming a lipid peroxy radical. This reaction may propagate the chain, leading to the formation of lipid peroxide (LOOH), which eventually can react further to yield malondialdehyde (MDA), a potent cross-linking agent. MDA has been hypothesized to cross-react with membrane lipids and proteins, rendering them incapable of performing their normal functions.

Because oxygen tension in the lens is low, free radical reactions may not involve molecular oxygen; instead, the free radicals may react directly with molecules. DNA is easily damaged by free radicals. Some of the damage to the lens is reparable, but some may be permanent. Free radicals can also attack the proteins or membrane lipids in the cortex. No repair mechanisms are known to ameliorate such damage, which increases with time. In lens fibers, where protein synthesis no longer takes place, free radical damage may lead to polymerization and cross-linking of lipids and proteins, resulting in an increase in the water-insoluble protein content.

The lens is equipped with several enzymes that protect against free radical or oxygen damage. These include glutathione peroxidase, catalase, and superoxide dismutase. Superoxide dismutase catalyzes the destruction of O_2 and produces hydrogen peroxide: $2O_2^- + 2H^+ \rightarrow H_2O_2 + O_2$. Catalase may break down the peroxide by the reaction: $2H_2O_2 \rightarrow 2H_2O + O_2$. Glutathione peroxidase catalyzes the reaction: $2GSH + LOOH \rightarrow GSSG + LOH + H_2O$. The glutathione disulfide (GSSG) is then reconverted to glutathione (GSH) by glutathione reductase, using the pyridine nucleotide NADPH provided by the HMP shunt as the reducing agent: $GSSG + NADPH + H^+ \rightarrow 2GSH + NADP^+$. Thus, glutathione acts indirectly as a major free radical scavenger in the lens.

Both vitamin E and ascorbic acid are present in the lens. Each of these substances can act as a free radical scavenger and thus protect against oxidative damage.

Andley UP, Liang JJN, Lou MF. Biochemical mechanisms of age-related cataract. In: Albert DM, Jakobiec FA, eds. *Principles and Practice of Ophthalmology.* 2nd ed. Philadelphia: Saunders; 2000:1428–1449.

Beebe DC. Lens. In: Kaufman PL, Alm A, eds. *Adler's Physiology of the Eye: Clinical Application.* 10th ed. St Louis: Mosby; 2003:117–158.

Jaffe NS, Horwitz J. Lens and cataract. In: Podos SM, Yanoff M, eds. *Textbook of Ophthalmology.* New York: Gower; 1992:vol. 3, ch 5, Evolution and molecular biology of lens proteins.

CHAPTER 3

Physiology

Throughout life, lens epithelial cells at the equator continue to divide and develop into lens fibers, resulting in continual growth of the lens. The area of the lens with the highest metabolic rate is the epithelium. Oxygen and glucose are utilized by the lens epithelium for protein synthesis and the active transport of electrolytes, carbohydrates, and amino acids into the lens. This chemical energy is required to maintain cell growth and transparency. Because the lens is avascular, the task of maintaining transparency faces several challenges. The aqueous humor functions as a source of nutrition and as a sink for lens waste products. However, only the anterior surface of the lens is bathed by the aqueous humor. The older cells, toward the center of the lens, must be able to communicate with the environment outside the lens. This communication is accomplished through low-resistance gap junctions that facilitate exchange from cell to cell.

Maintenance of Lens Water and Cation Balance

Perhaps the most important aspect of lens physiology is the mechanism that controls water and electrolyte balance, which is critical to lens transparency. Because lens transparency is highly dependent on the structural and macromolecular components, perturbation of cellular hydration can readily lead to opacification. It is noteworthy that disruption of water and electrolyte balance is not a feature of nuclear cataracts. In cortical cataracts, however, the water content rises significantly.

The normal human lens contains approximately 66% water and 33% protein, and this amount changes very little with aging. The lens cortex is more hydrated than the lens nucleus. About 5% of the lens volume is the water found between the lens fibers in the extracellular spaces. The sodium concentration in the lens is maintained at about 20 mM, and the potassium concentration is around 120 mM. Sodium and potassium levels in the surrounding aqueous humor and vitreous humor are quite different: sodium is much higher, about 150 mM, whereas potassium is approximately 5 mM.

Lens Epithelium: Site of Active Transport

The lens is dehydrated and has higher levels of potassium ions (K^+) and amino acids than the surrounding aqueous and vitreous. Conversely, the lens contains lower levels of sodium ions (Na^+), chloride ions (Cl^-), and water than the surrounding environment. The cation balance between the inside and outside of the lens is the result of both the permeability properties of the lens cell membranes and of the activity of the sodium pumps (Na^+,K^+-ATPase) that reside within the cell membranes of the lens epithelium and each lens fiber. The sodium pumps function by pumping sodium ions out while taking potassium ions in. This mechanism depends on ATP breakdown and is regulated by the enzyme Na^+,K^+-ATPase. This balance is easily disrupted by the specific ATPase inhibitor ouabain. Inhibition of Na^+,K^+-ATPase leads to loss of cation balance and elevated water content in the lens. Whether Na^+,K^+-ATPase is depressed in the development of cortical cataract is uncertain; some studies have shown reduced Na^+,K^+-ATPase activity, whereas others have shown no change. Still other studies have suggested that membrane permeability is increased with cataract development.

Pump-Leak Theory

The combination of active transport and membrane permeability is often referred to as the pump-leak system of the lens (Fig 3-1). According to the *pump-leak theory*, potassium and various other molecules such as amino acids are actively transported into the anterior lens via the epithelium. They then diffuse out with the concentration gradient through the back of the lens, where there are no active transport mechanisms. Conversely, sodium flows in through the back of the lens with a concentration gradient and then is actively exchanged for potassium by the epithelium. In support of this theory, an anteroposterior gradient was found for both ions: potassium was concentrated in the anterior lens and sodium was concentrated in the posterior lens. Conditions such as refrigeration that inactivate the energy-dependent enzyme pumps also abolish these gradients. Most of the Na^+,K^+-ATPase activity is found in the lens epithelium. The active transport mechanisms are lost if the capsule and attached epithelium are removed from the lens but not if the capsule alone is removed by enzymatic degradation with collagenase. These findings support the hypothesis that the epithelium is the primary site for active transport in the lens. Thus, sodium is pumped across the anterior face of the lens into the aqueous humor, and potassium moves from the aqueous humor into the lens. At the posterior surface of the lens (the lens–vitreous interface), the movement of solute occurs largely by passive diffusion. This asymmetric arrangement results in sodium and potassium gradients across the lens, with the concentration of potassium being higher at the front of the lens and lower at the back. Conversely, sodium concentration is higher at the back of the lens and lower at the front. Much of the diffusion throughout the lens occurs from cell to cell through the low-resistance gap junctions.

The unequal distribution of electrolytes across the lens cell membranes results in an electrical potential difference between the inside and outside of the lens. The inside of the lens is electronegative, measuring about –70 mV. There is even a –23-mV potential difference between the anterior and posterior surfaces of the lens. The normal potential difference of about 70 mV is readily altered by changes in pump activity or membrane permeability.

Calcium homeostasis is also critical to the lens. The normal intracellular level of calcium in the lens is about 30 mM, whereas the exterior calcium level is close to 2 μM. This large transmembrane calcium gradient is maintained primarily by the calcium pump (Ca^{2+}-ATPase). The lens cell membranes are also relatively impermeable to calcium. Loss of calcium homeostasis can be highly disruptive of lens metabolism. Increased levels

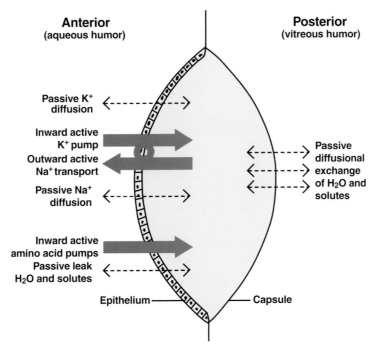

Anterior
(aqueous humor)

Posterior
(vitreous humor)

Passive K$^+$ diffusion

Inward active K$^+$ pump

Outward active Na$^+$ transport

Passive Na$^+$ diffusion

Inward active amino acid pumps

Passive leak H$_2$O and solutes

Passive diffusional exchange of H$_2$O and solutes

Epithelium

Capsule

Figure 3-1 The pump-leak hypothesis of pathways of solute movement in the lens. The major site of active transport mechanisms is in the anterior epithelium, whereas passive diffusion occurs over both surfaces. *(Modified with permission from Paterson CA, Delamere NA. The lens. In: Hart WM Jr, ed. Adler's Physiology of the Eye. 9th ed. St Louis: Mosby; 1992:365.)*

of calcium can result in many changes, including depressed glucose metabolism, formation of high-molecular-weight protein aggregates, and activation of destructive proteases.

Membrane transport and permeability are also important considerations in lens nutrition. Active amino acid transport takes place at the lens epithelium by a mechanism dependent on the sodium gradient, which is brought about by the sodium pump. Glucose enters the lens by a process of facilitated diffusion not directly linked to an active transport system. The waste products of lens metabolism leave the lens by simple diffusion. A variety of substances, including ascorbic acid, *myo*-inositol, and choline, have specialized transport mechanisms in the lens.

Accommodation

Accommodation, the mechanism by which the eye changes focus from distant to near images, is produced by a change in lens shape resulting from the action of the ciliary muscle on the zonular fibers. The lens substance is most malleable during childhood and the young adult years, progressively losing its ability to change shape with age. After approximately 40 years, the rigidity of the lens nucleus clinically reduces accommodation because the sclerotic nucleus cannot bulge anteriorly and change its anterior curvature as it could before.

According to the classic theory of von Helmholtz, most of the accommodative change in lens shape occurs at the central anterior lens surface. The central anterior capsule is thinner than the peripheral capsule (see Fig 1-3 in Chapter 1), and the anterior zonular fibers insert slightly closer to the visual axis than do the posterior zonular fibers, resulting in a central anterior bulge with accommodation. The posterior lens surface curvature changes minimally with accommodation. The central posterior capsule, which is the thinnest area of the capsule, tends to bulge posteriorly to the same extent regardless of zonular tension.

The ciliary muscle is a ring that, upon contraction, has the opposite effect from that intuitively expected of a sphincter. When a sphincter muscle contracts, it usually tightens its grip. However, when the ciliary muscle contracts, the diameter of the muscle ring is reduced, thereby relaxing the tension on the zonular fibers and allowing the lens to become more spherical. Thus, when the ciliary muscle contracts, the axial thickness of the lens increases, its diameter decreases, and its dioptric power increases, producing accommodation. When the ciliary muscle relaxes, the zonular tension increases, the lens flattens, and its dioptric power decreases (Table 3-1).

The accommodative response may be stimulated by the known or apparent size and distance of an object or by blur, chromatic aberration, or a continual oscillation of ciliary tone. Accommodation is mediated by the parasympathetic fibers of cranial nerve III (oculomotor). Parasympathomimetic drugs (eg, pilocarpine) induce accommodation, whereas parasympatholytic medications (eg, atropine) block accommodation. Drugs that relax the ciliary muscle are called *cycloplegics*.

The *amplitude of accommodation* is the amount of change in the eye's refractive power that is produced by accommodation. It diminishes with age and may be affected by some medications and diseases. Adolescents generally have 12–16 D of accommodation, whereas adults at age 40 have 4–8 D. After age 50, accommodation decreases to less than 2 D. It is thought that hardening of the lens with age is the principal cause of this loss of accommodation, which is called *presbyopia*. Research is under way into other possible contributing factors in presbyopia, such as changes in lens dimensions, in the elasticity of the lens capsule, and in the geometry of zonular attachments with age.

Glasser A, Kaufman PL. Accommodation and presbyopia. In: Kaufman PL, Alm A, eds. *Adler's Physiology of the Eye: Clinical Application.* 10th ed. St Louis: Mosby; 2003:197–233.

Table 3-1 Changes with Accommodation

	With Accommodation	Without Accommodation
Ciliary muscle action	Contraction	Relaxation
Ciliary ring diameter	Decreases	Increases
Zonular tension	Decreases	Increases
Lens shape	More spherical	Flatter
Lens equatorial diameter	Decreases	Increases
Axial lens thickness	Increases	Decreases
Central anterior lens capsule curvature	Steepens	Flattens
Central posterior lens capsule curvature	Minimal change	Minimal change
Lens dioptric power	Increases	Decreases

Presbyopia

Presbyopia is the loss of accommodation due to aging. According to von Helmholtz, as the crystalline lens ages, it becomes firmer and more sclerotic and resists deformation when the ciliary muscle contracts. Hence, it cannot bulge enough anteriorly to increase the lens curvature and dioptric power to focus at near.

Recently, an alternative theory of accommodation was hypothesized by Schachar based on increased equatorial growth of the lens. He proposed that, as the lens grows, lens fibers that resemble the rings on a tree are laid down at the equatorial zone. As the lens fibers accumulate within the capsular bag, the crystalline lens increases in size such that there is little or no room for lens movement with ciliary muscle contraction. If this theory is correct, increasing the ciliary space may allow for restored accommodation.

Schachar RA, Bax AJ. Mechanism of human accommodation as analyzed by nonlinear finite element analysis. *Compr Ther.* 2001;27:122–132.

Schachar RA, Cudmore DP, Black TD. Experimental support for Schachar's hypothesis of accommodation. *Ann Ophthalmol.* 1993;25:404–409.

This chapter was prepared with the assistance of Christopher A. Paterson, PhD, DSc.

CHAPTER 4

Embryology

Normal Development

The formation of the human crystalline lens begins very early in embryogenesis (Fig 4-1). At about 25 days of gestation, 2 lateral outpouchings called the *optic vesicles* form from the forebrain, or diencephalon. As the optic vesicles enlarge, they become closely apposed to the *surface ectoderm*, a single layer of cuboidal cells.

Lens Plate

The cells of the surface ectoderm that overlie the optic vesicles become columnar at about 27 days of gestation. This area of thickened cells is called the *lens plate*, or lens placode. A chemical mediator from the neuroectoderm is believed to stimulate the formation of the lens plate. Direct physical contact between surface ectoderm and neuroectoderm is not needed for this initial event in lens induction to occur.

Lens Pit

The *lens pit*, or *fovea lentis*, appears at 29 days of gestation as a small indentation inferior to the center of the lens plate. The lens pit deepens by a process of cellular multiplication and invaginates.

Lens Vesicle

As the lens pit continues to invaginate, the stalk of cells that connects it to the surface ectoderm constricts and eventually disappears. The resultant sphere, a single layer of cuboidal cells encased within a basement membrane (the *lens capsule*), is called the *lens vesicle*. At the time of its formation at 33 days of gestation, the lens vesicle is approximately 0.2 mm in diameter.

Because the lens vesicle was formed through a process of invagination of the surface ectoderm, the apices of the single layer of cells are oriented toward the lumen of the lens vesicle, with the base of each cell along the periphery of the vesicle. At the same time that the lens vesicle is forming, the optic vesicle is undergoing a process of invagination as it begins to form the 2-layered *optic cup*.

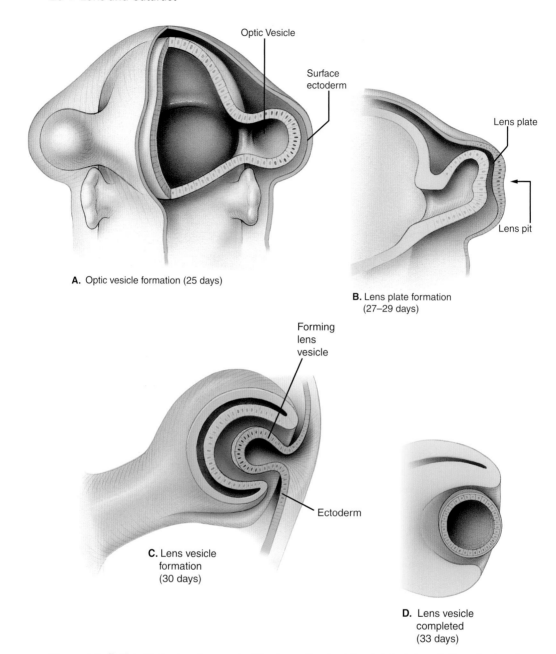

Figure 4-1 Embryologic development of the lens. See text for detailed description of artwork. *(Illustration by Christine Gralapp.)* *(Continues on next page.)*

Primary Lens Fibers and the Embryonic Nucleus

The posterior cells of the lens vesicle become more columnar and begin to elongate. As these cells elongate, they progressively obliterate the lumen of the lens vesicle. At approximately 40 days of gestation, the lumen of the lens vesicle is completely obliterated. The elongated cells are called the *primary lens fibers*. The nuclei of the primary lens fibers

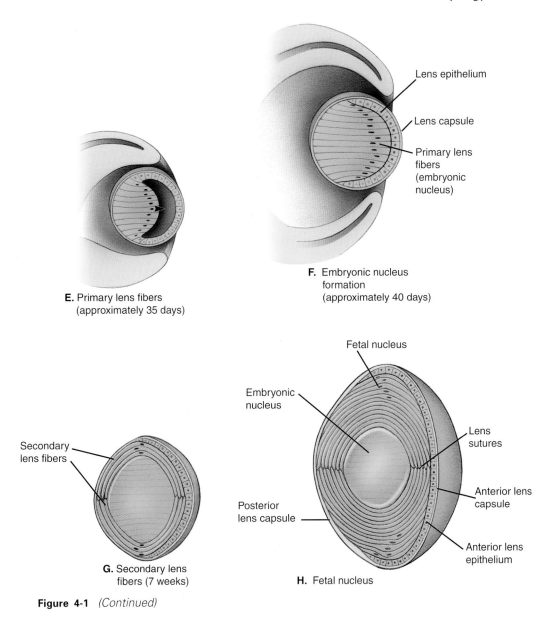

Lens epithelium

Lens capsule

Primary lens fibers (embryonic nucleus)

F. Embryonic nucleus formation (approximately 40 days)

E. Primary lens fibers (approximately 35 days)

Fetal nucleus

Embryonic nucleus

Secondary lens fibers

Lens sutures

Posterior lens capsule

Anterior lens capsule

Anterior lens epithelium

G. Secondary lens fibers (7 weeks)

H. Fetal nucleus

Figure 4-1 *(Continued)*

move from near the posterior basal lamina to a position more anterior within the lens fibers and subsequently become pyknotic as the intracellular organelles become indistinct. The primary lens fibers make up the *embryonic nucleus* that will ultimately occupy the central area of the lens in adult life.

Although the cells of the posterior layer of the optic vesicle undergo marked differentiation to form the primary lens fibers, the cells of the anterior lens vesicle do not change. This monolayer of cuboidal cells is now referred to as the *lens epithelium*. Subsequent differentiation and growth of the lens originates from the lens epithelium. The *lens capsule* develops as a basement membrane elaborated by the lens epithelium anteriorly and by lens fibers posteriorly.

Secondary Lens Fibers

At about 7 weeks of gestation, the cells of the lens epithelium in the area of the equator begin to multiply rapidly and elongate to form *secondary lens fibers.* The anterior aspect of each developing lens fiber grows anteriorly toward the anterior pole of the lens, insinuating itself underneath the lens epithelium. The posterior aspect of each developing lens fiber grows posteriorly toward the posterior pole of the lens, just inside the lens capsule. In this manner, new lens fibers are continually formed, layer upon layer. The secondary lens fibers formed between 2 and 8 months of gestation make up the *fetal nucleus.*

Lens Sutures and the Fetal Nucleus

As lens fibers grow anteriorly and posteriorly, a pattern emerges where the fibers meet and interdigitate in the anterior and posterior portions of the lens. These patterns are known as *sutures.* Y-shaped sutures are recognizable at about 8 weeks of gestation, with an erect Y-suture appearing anteriorly and an inverted Y-suture posteriorly (Fig 4-2).

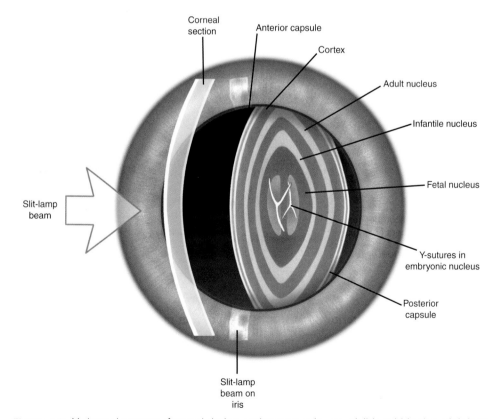

Figure 4-2 Y-shaped sutures, formed during embryogenesis, are visible within the adult lens with the slit lamp. *(Illustration by Christine Gralapp.)*

Only during fetal life are Y-sutures formed. As the lens fibers continue to form and the lens continues to grow, the pattern of lens sutures becomes increasingly complex.

At birth, the human lens weighs approximately 90 mg, and it increases in mass at the rate of about 2 mg per year as new fibers form. After 20 years, the central, or oldest, lens fibers become less malleable and the lens nucleus becomes more rigid. After 40 years, the rigidity of the lens nucleus clinically reduces accommodation, and by age 60 nuclear sclerosis or discoloration often makes the lens sutures difficult to distinguish.

Tunica Vasculosa Lentis

As the lens develops, a nutritive support structure, the *tunica vasculosa lentis* (Fig 4-3), forms around it. At about 1 month of gestation, the hyaloid artery gives rise to small capillaries that form an anastomotic net covering the posterior aspect of the developing lens. This *posterior vascular capsule* branches into small capillaries that then grow toward the equator of the lens, where they anastomose with choroidal veins and form the *capsulopupillary portion* of the tunica vasculosa lentis. Branches of the long ciliary arteries anastomose with branches of the capsulopupillary portion to form the *anterior vascular capsule*, sometimes called the *pupillary membrane*, which covers the anterior surface of the lens.

The anterior vascular capsule is fully developed at approximately 9 weeks of gestation and disappears shortly before birth. Sometimes a remnant of the posterior vascular capsule persists as a *Mittendorf dot*, a small opacity or strand on the posterior aspect of the

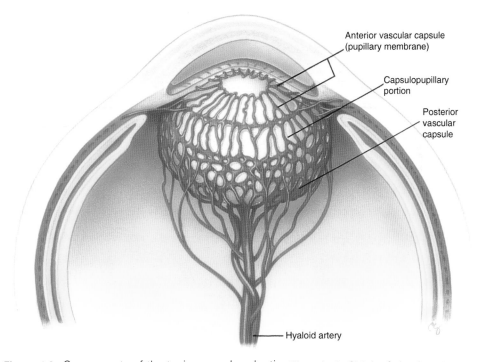

Anterior vascular capsule (pupillary membrane)

Capsulopupillary portion

Posterior vascular capsule

Hyaloid artery

Figure 4-3 Components of the tunica vasculosa lentis. *(Illustration by Christine Gralapp.)*

lens in normal adult eyes. Remnants of the anterior vascular capsule are often visible in young healthy eyes as pupillary strands.

Zonules of Zinn

Experimental evidence suggests that the zonular fibers are secreted by the ciliary epithelium. The zonular fibers begin to develop at the end of the third month of gestation.

Duke-Elder S, ed. *System of Ophthalmology*. St Louis: Mosby; 1973; 4:127–137.

Kuszak JR, Clark JI, Cooper KE, et al. Biology of the lens: lens transparency as a function of embryology, anatomy, and physiology. In: Albert DM, Jakobiec FA, eds. *Principles and Practice of Ophthalmology*. 2nd ed. Philadelphia: Saunders; 2000:1355–1408.

Kuszak JR, Costello MJ. Embryology and anatomy of human lenses. In: Tasman W, Jaeger EA, eds. *Duane's Clinical Ophthalmology*. Philadelphia: Lippincott; 2002:vol 1, ch 71A:1–20.

Streeten BW. Zonular apparatus; Worgul BV. The lens. In: Jakobiec FA, ed. *Ocular Anatomy, Embryology, and Teratology*. Philadelphia: Harper & Row; 1982:331–353.

Congenital Anomalies and Abnormalities

Congenital Aphakia

The lens is absent in *congenital aphakia*, a very rare anomaly. Two forms of congenital aphakia have been described. In *primary aphakia*, the lens plate fails to form from the surface ectoderm in the developing embryo. *Secondary aphakia*, the more common type, occurs when the developing lens is spontaneously absorbed. Both primary and secondary aphakia are usually associated with other malformations of the eye.

Lenticonus and Lentiglobus

Lenticonus is a localized, cone-shaped deformation of the anterior or posterior lens surface (Fig 4-4). Posterior lenticonus is more common than anterior lenticonus and is usually unilateral and axial in location. Anterior lenticonus, which is often bilateral, may be associated with Alport syndrome.

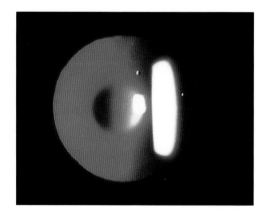

Figure 4-4 Posterior lenticonus as viewed by retroillumination.

In *lentiglobus,* the localized deformation of the lens surface is spherical. Posterior lentiglobus is more common than anterior lentiglobus and is often associated with posterior pole opacities that vary in density.

Retinoscopy through the center of the lens reveals a distorted and myopic reflex in both lenticonus and lentiglobus. These deformations can also be seen in the red reflex, where they appear as an "oil droplet" by retroillumination. (This condition should not be confused with the "oil droplet" cataract of galactosemia, which is discussed in Chapter 5.) The posterior bulging may progress with initial worsening of the myopia, followed by opacification of the defect. Surrounding cortical lamellae may also opacify.

Lens Coloboma

A *lens coloboma* is an anomaly of lens shape (Fig 4-5). Lens colobomas may be classified into 2 types: *primary coloboma,* a wedge-shaped defect or indentation of the lens periphery that occurs as an isolated anomaly; and *secondary coloboma,* a flattening or indentation of the lens periphery caused by the lack of ciliary body or zonular development. Lens colobomas are typically located inferiorly and may be associated with colobomas of the uvea. Cortical lens opacification or thickening of the lens capsule may appear adjacent to the coloboma. The zonular attachments in the region of the coloboma usually show some defect.

Mittendorf Dot

Mittendorf dot, or hyaloid corpuscle, is a common anomaly observed in many healthy eyes. A small, dense white spot generally located inferonasal to the posterior pole of the lens, a Mittendorf dot is a remnant of the posterior vascular capsule of the tunica vasculosa lentis. It marks the place where the hyaloid artery came into contact with the posterior surface of the lens in utero. Sometimes a Mittendorf dot is associated with a fibrous tail or remnant of the hyaloid artery projecting into the vitreous body.

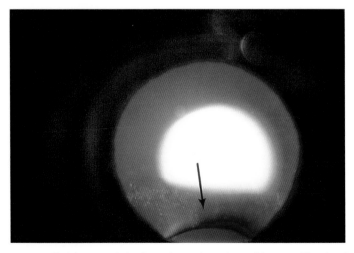

Figure 4-5 Coloboma of the lens *(arrow)* as viewed by retroillumination.

Epicapsular Star

Another very common remnant of the tunica vasculosa lentis is an *epicapsular star* (Fig 4-6). It consists of a star-shaped distribution of tiny brown or golden flecks, often called chicken tracks, on the central anterior lens capsule.

Peters Anomaly

Historically called posterior corneal defect, *Peters anomaly* is part of a spectrum of disorders known as *anterior segment dysgenesis syndrome,* also known as neurocristopathy and mesodermal dysgenesis. Peters anomaly is characterized by a central or paracentral corneal opacity (leukoma) associated with the thinning or absence of adjacent endothelium and Descemet's membrane. Patients with Peters anomaly may also display the following lens anomalies:

- adhesions between lens and cornea
- anterior cortical or polar cataract
- a misshapen lens displaced anteriorly into the pupillary space and the anterior chamber
- microspherophakia

Microspherophakia

Microspherophakia is a developmental abnormality in which the lens is small in diameter and spherical in shape. The entire lens equator can be visualized at the slit lamp when the pupil is widely dilated (Fig 4-7). As a result of the increased refractive power of the spherical shape of the lens, the eye is highly myopic.

Faulty development of the secondary lens fibers during embryogenesis is believed to be the cause of microspherophakia. This condition may occur as an isolated hereditary abnormality or occasionally in association with Peters anomaly, Marfan syndrome, Alport

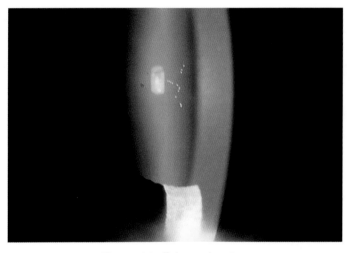

Figure 4-6 Epicapsular star.

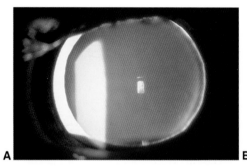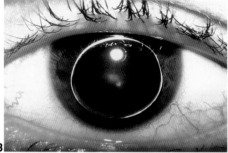

A   B

Figure 4-7 Microspherophakia. **A**, When the pupil is dilated, the entire lens equator can be seen at the slit lamp. **B**, Anterior dislocation of a microspherophakic lens. *(Part A courtesy of Karla J. Johns, MD.)*

syndrome, Lowe syndrome, or congenital rubella. However, microspherophakia is most often seen as a part of Weill-Marchesani syndrome. People with Weill-Marchesani syndrome commonly have small stature, short and stubby fingers, and broad hands with reduced joint mobility. Weill-Marchesani syndrome is usually inherited as an autosomal recessive trait.

The spherically shaped lens can block the pupil and cause angle-closure glaucoma. Miotics aggravate this condition by increasing pupillary block and allowing further forward displacement of the lens. Cycloplegics are the medical treatment of choice to break an attack of angle-closure glaucoma in patients with microspherophakia because they decrease pupillary block by tightening the zonular fibers, decreasing the anteroposterior lens diameter, and pulling the lens posteriorly. A laser iridotomy may also be useful in relieving angle closure in patients with microspherophakia. (See also BCSC Section 10, *Glaucoma.*)

Aniridia

Aniridia is an uncommon panocular syndrome in which the most dramatic manifestation is partial or nearly complete absence of the iris (Fig 4-8). Associated findings include corneal pannus and epitheliopathy, glaucoma, foveal and optic nerve hypoplasia, and nystagmus. Aniridia is almost always bilateral. Two thirds of cases are familial and one third are sporadic. Sporadic cases of aniridia are associated with a high incidence of Wilms tumor and the WAGR complex (Wilms tumor, aniridia, genitourinary malformations, and mental retardation).

Anterior and posterior polar lens opacities may be present at birth in patients with aniridia. Cortical, subcapsular, and lamellar opacities develop in 50%–85% of patients within the first 2 decades. The lens opacities may progress and further impair vision. Poor zonular integrity and ectopia lentis have also been reported in patients with aniridia.

Congenital and Infantile Cataract

The term *congenital cataract* refers to a lens opacity present at birth. Lens opacities that develop during the first year of life are called *infantile cataracts*. Because some lens opacities escape detection at birth and are noted only on later examination, these terms are

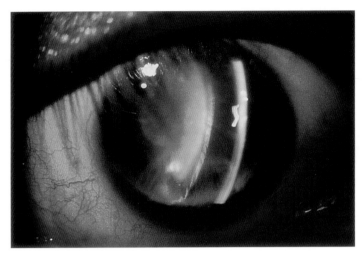

Figure 4-8 Cataract in aniridic patient.

used interchangeably by many physicians. Congenital and infantile cataracts are fairly common, occurring in 1 out of every 2000 live births. Congenital and infantile cataracts cover a broad spectrum of severity: whereas some lens opacities do not progress and are visually insignificant, others can produce profound visual impairment.

Congenital and infantile cataracts may be unilateral or bilateral. They can be classified by morphology, presumed etiology, presence of specific metabolic disorders, or associated ocular anomalies or systemic findings (Table 4-1). In general, about one third of congenital or infantile cataracts are associated with other disease syndromes, one third occur as an inherited trait, and one third result from undetermined causes. Metabolic diseases tend to be more commonly associated with bilateral cataracts. (For a discussion of the systemic evaluation of patients with congenital cataracts, see BCSC Section 6, *Pediatric Ophthalmology and Strabismus*.)

Morphologic Classification of Congenital and Infantile Cataracts

Congenital cataracts occur in a variety of morphologic configurations, including polar, sutural, coronary, cerulean, nuclear, capsular, lamellar, complete, and membranous. Each of these categories encompasses a range of severity.

Polar *AD*

Polar cataracts are lens opacities that involve the subcapsular cortex and lens capsule of the anterior or posterior pole of the lens (Fig 4-9). *Anterior polar cataracts* are usually small, bilateral, symmetric, nonprogressive opacities that do not impair vision. They are frequently inherited in an autosomal dominant pattern. Anterior polar cataracts are sometimes seen in association with other ocular abnormalities, including microphthalmos, persistent pupillary membrane, and anterior lenticonus.

Posterior polar cataracts generally produce more visual impairment than do anterior polar cataracts because they tend to be larger and are positioned closer to the nodal point

Table 4-1 Etiology of Pediatric Cataracts

Bilateral cataracts
Idiopathic
Hereditary cataracts (autosomal dominant most common, also autosomal recessive or X-linked)
Genetic and metabolic diseases
   Down syndrome
   Hallermann-Streiff syndrome
   Lowe syndrome
   Galactosemia
   Marfan syndrome
   Trisomy 13–15
   Hypoglycemia
   Alport syndrome
   Myotonic dystrophy
   Fabry disease
   Hypoparathyroidism
   Conradi syndrome
Maternal infection
   Rubella
   Cytomegalovirus
   Varicella
   Syphilis
   Toxoplasmosis
Ocular anomalies
   Aniridia
   Anterior segment dysgenesis syndrome
Toxic
   Corticosteroids
   Radiation (may also be unilateral)

Unilateral cataracts
Idiopathic
Ocular anomalies
   Persistent fetal vasculature (PFV)
   Anterior segment dysgenesis
   Posterior lenticonus
   Posterior pole tumors
Traumatic (rule out child abuse)
Rubella
Masked bilateral cataract

of the eye. Capsular fragility has been reported. Posterior polar cataracts are usually stable but occasionally progress. They may be sporadic or familial. Familial posterior polar cataracts are usually bilateral and inherited in an autosomal dominant pattern. Sporadic posterior polar cataracts are often unilateral and may be associated with remnants of the tunica vasculosa lentis or with an abnormality of the posterior capsule such as lenticonus or lentiglobus.

Sutural AD

The *sutural, or stellate, cataract* is an opacification of the Y-sutures of the fetal nucleus that usually does not impair vision (Fig 4-10). These opacities often have branches or

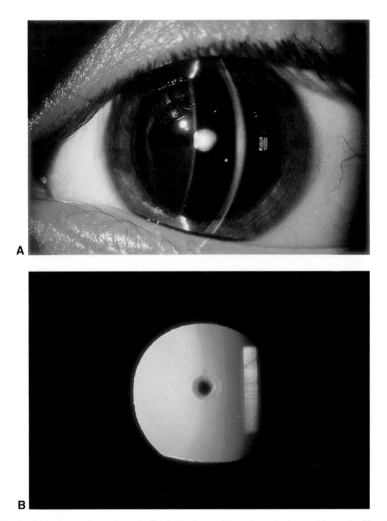

Figure 4-9 **A**, Anterior polar cataract. **B**, Anterior polar cataract viewed by retroillumination.

knobs projecting from them. Bilateral and symmetric, sutural cataracts are frequently inherited in an autosomal dominant pattern.

Coronary AD

Coronary cataracts are so named because they consist of a group of club-shaped opacities in the cortex that are arranged around the equator of the lens like a crown, or *corona*. They cannot be seen unless the pupil is dilated, and they usually do not affect visual acuity. Coronary cataracts are often inherited in an autosomal dominant pattern.

Cerulean

Also known as blue-dot cataracts, *cerulean cataracts* are small bluish opacities located in the lens cortex (Fig 4-11). They are nonprogressive and usually do not cause visual symptoms.

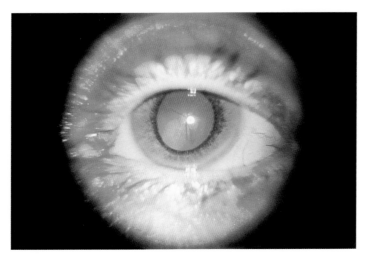

Figure 4-10 Sutural cataract.

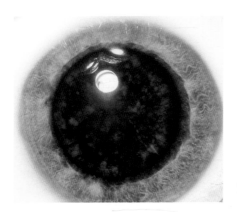

Figure 4-11 A cerulean cataract consists of small bluish opacities in the cortex. *(Photograph courtesy of Karla J. Johns, MD.)*

Nuclear

Congenital nuclear cataracts are opacities of either the embryonic nucleus alone or both the embryonic and fetal nuclei (Fig 4-12). They are usually bilateral, with a wide spectrum of severity. Lens opacification may involve the complete nucleus or be limited to discrete layers within the nucleus. Eyes with congenital nuclear cataracts tend to be small.

Capsular

Capsular cataracts are small opacifications of the lens epithelium and anterior lens capsule that spare the cortex. They are differentiated from anterior polar cataracts by their protrusion into the anterior chamber. Capsular cataracts generally do not adversely affect vision.

Lamellar AD

Lamellar, or *zonular, cataracts* are the most common type of congenital/infantile cataract (Fig 4-13). They are characteristically bilateral and symmetric, and their effect on visual

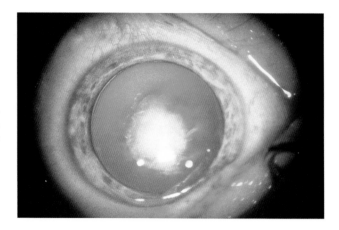

Figure 4-12 Congenital nuclear cataract. *(Reproduced from Day SH.* Understanding and Preventing Amblyopia. Eye Care Skills for the Primary Care Physician Series *[slide-script]. San Francisco: American Academy of Ophthalmology; 1987.)*

acuity varies with the size and density of the opacity. In some cases, lamellar cataracts may be the result of a transient toxic influence during embryogenic lens development. The earlier this toxic influence occurs, the smaller and deeper is the resulting lamellar cataract. Lamellar cataracts may also be inherited as an autosomal dominant trait.

Lamellar cataracts are opacifications of specific layers or zones of the lens. Clinically, the cataract is visible as an opacified layer that surrounds a clearer center and is itself surrounded by a layer of clear cortex. Viewed from the front, the lamellar cataract has a disk-shaped configuration. Often, additional arcuate opacities within the cortex straddle the equator of the lamellar cataract; these horseshoe-shaped opacities are called *riders*.

Complete

With *complete*, or *total*, *cataract*, all of the lens fibers are opacified. The red reflex is completely obscured, and the retina cannot be seen with either direct or indirect ophthalmoscopy. Some cataracts may be subtotal at birth and progress rapidly to become complete cataracts. Complete cataracts may be unilateral or bilateral and produce profound visual impairment.

Membranous

Membranous cataracts occur when lens proteins are resorbed from either an intact or traumatized lens, allowing the anterior and posterior lens capsules to fuse into a dense white membrane (Fig 4-14). The resulting opacity and lens distortion generally cause significant visual disability.

Rubella

Maternal infection with the rubella virus, an RNA togavirus, can cause fetal damage, especially if the infection occurs during the first trimester of pregnancy. Systemic manifestations of congenital rubella infection include cardiac defects, deafness, and mental retardation.

Cataracts resulting from *congenital rubella syndrome* are characterized by pearly white nuclear opacifications. Sometimes the entire lens is opacified (complete cataract), and the cortex may liquefy. Histopathologically, lens fiber nuclei are retained deep within the

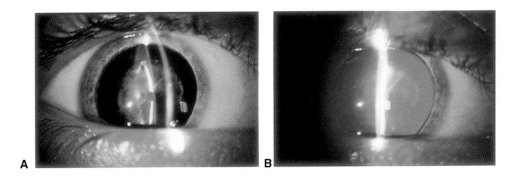

A   B

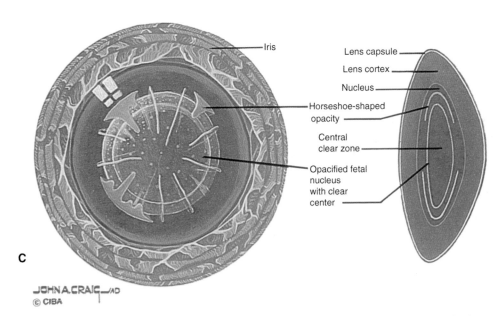

Iris

Lens capsule
Lens cortex
Nucleus
Horseshoe-shaped opacity
Central clear zone
Opacified fetal nucleus with clear center

C

JOHN A. CRAIG—MD
© CIBA

Figure 4-13 **A**, Lamellar cataract. **B**, Lamellar cataract viewed by retroillumination. **C**, Schematic of lamellar cataract. *(Courtesy of CIBA Pharmaceutical Co., division of CIBA-GEIGY Corp. Reproduced with permission from* Clinical Symposia. *Illustration by John A. Craig.)*

lens substance. Live virus particles may be recovered from the lens as late as 3 years after the patient's birth. Cataract removal may be complicated by excessive postoperative inflammation caused by release of these live virus particles.

Other ocular manifestations of congenital rubella syndrome include diffuse pigmentary retinopathy, microphthalmos, glaucoma, and transient or permanent corneal clouding. Although congenital rubella syndrome may cause cataract or glaucoma, both conditions are usually not present simultaneously in the same eye.

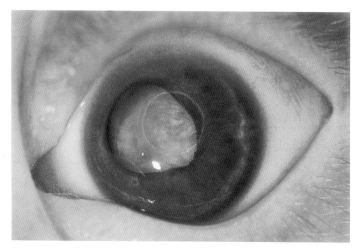

Figure 4-14 Membranous cataract.

Developmental Defects

Ectopia Lentis

Ectopia lentis is a displacement of the lens that may be congenital, developmental, or acquired. A *subluxated* lens is partially displaced from its normal position but remains in the pupillary area. A *luxated,* or *dislocated,* lens is completely displaced from the pupil, implying separation of all zonular attachments. Findings associated with lens subluxation include decreased vision, marked astigmatism, monocular diplopia, and iridodonesis (tremulous iris). Potential complications of ectopia lentis include cataract and displacement of the lens into the anterior chamber or into the vitreous. Dislocation into the anterior chamber or pupil may cause pupillary block and angle-closure glaucoma. Dislocation of the lens posteriorly into the vitreous cavity often has no adverse sequelae.

Trauma is the most common cause of acquired lens displacement. Nontraumatic ectopia lentis is commonly associated with Marfan syndrome, homocystinuria, aniridia, and congenital glaucoma. Less frequently, it appears with Ehlers-Danlos syndrome, hyperlysinemia, and sulfite oxidase deficiency. Ectopia lentis may occur as an isolated anomaly (simple ectopia lentis), usually inherited as an autosomal dominant trait. Ectopia lentis can also be associated with pupillary abnormalities in the ocular syndrome ectopia lentis et pupillae (see Developmental Defects, Ectopia Lentis et Pupillae).

Marfan Syndrome

Marfan syndrome is a heritable disorder with ocular, cardiac, and skeletal manifestations. Although usually inherited as an autosomal dominant trait, the disorder appears with no family history in about 15% of cases. Marfan syndrome is believed to result from an abnormality of fibrillin, a connective tissue component. Affected individuals are tall, with arachnodactyly (Fig 4-15A) and chest wall deformities. Associated cardiac abnormalities include dilated aortic root and mitral valve prolapse.

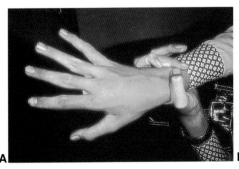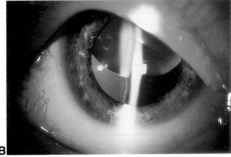

Figure 4-15 Marfan syndrome. **A**, Arachnodactyly in a patient with Marfan syndrome. **B**, Subluxated lens in Marfan syndrome. *(Part A courtesy of Karla J. Johns, MD.)*

From 50% to 80% of patients with Marfan syndrome exhibit ectopia lentis (Fig 4-15B). The lens subluxation tends to be bilateral and symmetric (usually superior and temporal), but variations do occur. The zonular attachments commonly remain intact but become stretched and elongated. Ectopia lentis in Marfan syndrome is probably congenital in most cases. Progression of lens subluxation is observed in some patients over time, whereas in many patients the lens position remains stable.

Ocular abnormalities associated with Marfan syndrome include axial myopia and an increased risk of retinal detachment. Patients with Marfan syndrome may develop pupillary block glaucoma if the lens dislocates into the pupil or anterior chamber. Open-angle glaucoma may also occur. In addition, children with lens subluxation may develop amblyopia if their refractive error shows significant asymmetry or remains uncorrected in early childhood.

Spectacle or contact lens correction of the refractive error provides satisfactory visual acuity in most cases. Pupillary dilation is sometimes helpful. Both the phakic and aphakic portions of the pupil may be refracted to determine the optimum visual acuity. A reading add is often necessary because the subluxated lens lacks sufficient accommodation.

In some cases, adequate visual acuity cannot be obtained with spectacle or contact lens correction, and removal of the lens may be indicated. Lens extraction—either extracapsular or intracapsular—in patients with Marfan syndrome is associated with a high rate of complications such as vitreous loss and complicated retinal detachment. (Intracapsular and extracapsular cataract extraction are discussed in detail in Chapter 8.) Recently, improved results have been reported with lensectomy using vitrectomy instrumentation, although the long-term results are not yet known.

Homocystinuria

Homocystinuria is an autosomal recessive disorder, an inborn error of methionine metabolism. Serum levels of homocystine and methionine are elevated. Affected individuals are normal at birth but develop seizures, osteoporosis, and mental retardation. They are usually tall with light-colored hair. Patients with homocystinuria are also prone to thromboembolic episodes, and surgery and general anesthesia are thought to increase the risk of thromboembolism.

Lens dislocation in homocystinuria tends to be bilateral and symmetric. Lens dislocation appears in infancy in about 30% of affected individuals, and by the age of 15 years it appears in 80% of those affected. The lenses are usually subluxated inferiorly and nasally, but variations have been reported. Because zonular fibers of the lens are known to have a high concentration of cysteine, deficiency of cysteine is thought to disturb normal zonular development; affected fibers tend to be brittle and easily disrupted. Studies of infants with homocystinuria treated with a low-methionine, high-cysteine diet and vitamin supplementation with the coenzyme pyridoxine (vitamin B_6) have shown promise in reducing the incidence of ectopia lentis.

Hyperlysinemia

Hyperlysinemia, an inborn error of metabolism of the amino acid lysine, is associated with ectopia lentis. Affected individuals also show mental retardation and muscular hypotony.

Sulfite Oxidase Deficiency

Sulfite oxidase deficiency is a very rare autosomal recessive metabolic disorder of sulfur metabolism. In addition to ectopia lentis, other manifestations include severe mental retardation and seizures.

Ectopia Lentis et Pupillae

In the autosomal recessive disorder *ectopia lentis et pupillae*, the lens and the pupil are displaced in opposite directions. The pupil is irregular, usually slit shaped, and displaced from the normal position. The dislocated lens may bisect the pupil or may be completely luxated from the pupillary space. This disorder is usually bilateral but not symmetric. Characteristically, the iris dilates poorly. Associated ocular anomalies include severe axial myopia, retinal detachment, enlarged corneal diameter, cataract, and abnormal iris transillumination.

Persistent Fetal Vasculature

Persistent fetal vasculature (PFV), also known as *persistent hyperplastic primary vitreous (PHPV)*, is a congenital, nonhereditary ocular malformation that frequently involves the lens. A white, fibrous, retrolental tissue is present, often in association with posterior cortical opacification. Progressive cataract formation often occurs, sometimes leading to a complete cataract. Other abnormalities associated with PFV include elongation of the ciliary processes, prominent radial iris vessels, and persistent hyaloid artery. PFV is usually unilateral. (See also BCSC Section 6, *Pediatric Ophthalmology and Strabismus;* and Section 12, *Retina and Vitreous.*)

Gold DH, Weingeist TA, eds. *The Eye in Systemic Disease.* Philadelphia: Lippincott; 1990:309–414, 513–580.

Goldberg MF. Persistent fetal vasculature (PFV): an integrated interpretation of signs and symptoms associated with persistent hyperplastic primary vitreous (PHPV). LIV Edward Jackson Memorial Lecture. *Am J Ophthalmol.* 1997;124:587–626.

Hiles DA, Kilty LA. Disorders of the lens. In: Isenberg SJ, ed. *The Eye in Infancy.* 2nd ed. St
Louis: Mosby; 1994:336–373.

Jaffe NS, Horwitz J. Lens alterations. In: Podos SM, Yanoff M, eds. *Textbook of Ophthalmology.*
Vol 3. New York: Gower; 1992: chap 8, pp 8.1–8.16.

Lambert S. Lens. In: Taylor D, ed. *Paediatric Ophthalmology.* 2nd ed. Boston: Blackwell Science; 1997:445–476.

Nelson LB, Maumenee IH. Ectopia lentis. *Surv Ophthalmol.* 1982;27:143–160.

Streeten BW. Pathology of the lens. In: Albert DM, Jakobiec FA, eds. *Principles and Practice
of Ophthalmology.* 2nd ed. Philadelphia: Saunders; 2000;4:3685–3749.

CHAPTER 5

Pathology

Aging Changes

Age-related cataract is a very common cause of visual impairment in older adults. The pathogenesis of age-related cataracts is multifactorial and not completely understood. As the lens ages, it increases in weight and thickness and decreases in accommodative power. As new layers of cortical fibers are formed concentrically, the lens nucleus undergoes compression and hardening (nuclear sclerosis). Crystallins (lens proteins) are changed by chemical modification and aggregation into high-molecular-weight protein. The resulting protein aggregates cause abrupt fluctuations in the refractive index of the lens, scatter light rays, and reduce transparency. Chemical modification of nuclear lens proteins also produces progressive pigmentation. The lens takes on a yellow or brownish hue with advancing age (Fig 5-1). Other age-related changes in the lens include decreased concentrations of glutathione and potassium and increased concentrations of sodium and calcium.

The 3 main types of age-related cataracts are nuclear, cortical, and posterior subcapsular cataracts. In many patients, components of more than one type are present. (See also BCSC Section 4, *Ophthalmic Pathology and Intraocular Tumors.*)

Nuclear Cataracts

Some degree of nuclear sclerosis and yellowing is considered physiologically normal in adult patients past middle age. In general, this condition interferes only minimally with visual function. An excessive amount of sclerosis and yellowing is called a *nuclear cataract*, which causes a central opacity (Fig 5-2). The degree of sclerosis, yellowing, and opacification is evaluated with a slit-lamp biomicroscope and by examining the red reflex with the pupil dilated.

Nuclear cataracts tend to progress slowly. Although they are usually bilateral, they may be asymmetric. Nuclear cataracts typically cause greater impairment of distance vision than of near vision. In the early stages, the progressive hardening of the lens nucleus frequently causes an increase in the refractive index of the lens and thus a myopic shift in refraction (*lenticular myopia*). In some cases, the myopic shift enables otherwise presbyopic individuals to read without spectacles, a condition referred to as *second sight*. Occasionally, the abrupt change in refractive index between the sclerotic nucleus (or other lens opacities) and the lens cortex can cause monocular diplopia. Progressive yellowing of the lens causes poor hue discrimination, especially at the blue end of the visible light

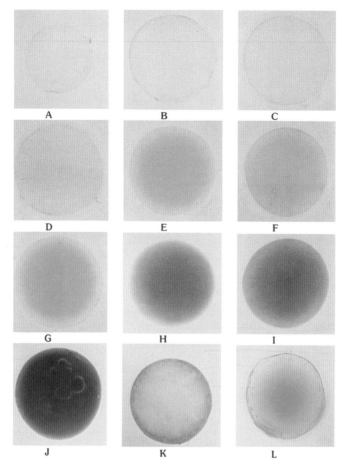

Figure 5-1 Increasing yellow-to-brown coloration of the human lens from 6 months **(A)** through 8 years **(B)**, 12 years **(C)**, 25 years **(D)**, 47 years **(E)**, 60 years **(F)**, 70 years **(G)**, 82 years **(H)**, and 91 years **(I)**. Brown nuclear cataract in 70-year-old patient **(J)**, cortical cataract in 68-year-old **(K)**, and mixed nuclear and cortical cataract in 74-year-old **(L)**. *(Reproduced with permission from Lerman S. Phototoxicity: clinical considerations.* Focal Points: Clinical Modules for Ophthalmologists. *San Francisco: American Academy of Ophthalmology; 1987, module 8.)*

spectrum. Photopic retinal function may decrease with advanced nuclear cataract. In very advanced cases, the lens nucleus becomes opaque and brown and is called a *brunescent* nuclear cataract.

Histopathologically, nuclear cataracts are characterized by homogeneity of the lens nucleus with loss of cellular laminations.

Cortical Cataracts

Changes in the ionic composition of the lens cortex and subsequent changes in hydration of the lens fibers lead to cortical opacification. *Cortical cataracts* are usually bilateral but are often asymmetric. Their effect on visual function varies greatly, depending on the location of the opacification relative to the visual axis. A common symptom of cortical

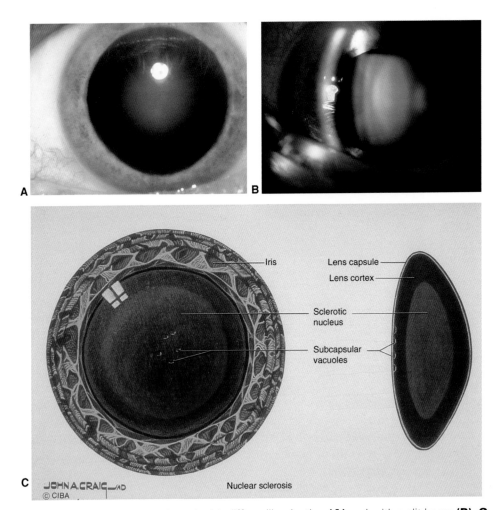

Figure 5-2 Nuclear cataract viewed with diffuse illumination **(A)** and with a slit beam **(B)**. **C,** Schematic of nuclear cataract. *(Courtesy of CIBA Pharmaceutical Co., division of CIBA-GEIGY Corp. Reproduced with permission from Clinical Symposia. Illustration by John A. Craig.)*

cataracts is glare from intense focal light sources, such as car headlights. Monocular diplopia may also result. Cortical cataracts vary greatly in their rate of progression; some cortical opacities remain unchanged for prolonged periods, whereas others progress rapidly.

The first signs of cortical cataract formation visible with the slit-lamp biomicroscope are vacuoles and water clefts in the anterior or posterior cortex (Fig 5-3). The cortical lamellae may be separated by fluid. Wedge-shaped opacities (often called *cortical spokes* or *cuneiform opacities*) form near the periphery of the lens, with the pointed end of the opacities oriented toward the center (Fig 5-4). The cortical spokes appear as white opacities when viewed with the slit-lamp biomicroscope and as dark shadows when viewed by retroillumination. The wedge-shaped opacities may enlarge and coalesce to form large

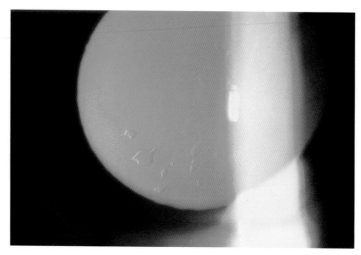

Figure 5-3 Vacuoles in early cortical cataract development.

cortical opacities. As the lens continues to take up water, it may swell and become an *intumescent* cortical cataract. When the entire cortex from the capsule to the nucleus becomes white and opaque, the cataract is said to be *mature* (Fig 5-5).

A *hypermature* cataract occurs when degenerated cortical material leaks through the lens capsule, leaving the capsule wrinkled and shrunken (Fig 5-6). A *morgagnian* cataract occurs when further liquefaction of the cortex allows free movement of the nucleus within the capsular bag (Fig 5-7).

Histopathologically, cortical cataracts are characterized by hydropic swelling of the lens fibers. Globules of eosinophilic material (morgagnian globules) are observed in slit-like spaces between lens fibers.

Posterior Subcapsular Cataracts

Posterior subcapsular cataracts (PSCs) are often seen in patients younger than those presenting with nuclear or cortical cataracts. PSCs are located in the posterior cortical layer and are usually axial (Fig 5-8). The first indication of PSC formation is a subtle iridescent sheen in the posterior cortical layers visible with the slit lamp. In later stages, granular opacities and a plaquelike opacity of the posterior subcapsular cortex appear.

The patient often complains of glare and poor vision under bright lighting conditions because the PSC obscures more of the pupillary aperture when miosis is induced by bright lights, accommodation, or miotics. Near visual acuity tends to be reduced more than distance visual acuity. Some patients experience monocular diplopia. Slit-lamp detection of PSCs can best be accomplished through a dilated pupil. Retroillumination is also helpful.

In addition to being one of the main types of age-related cataract, PSCs can occur as a result of trauma, systemic or topical corticosteroid use, inflammation, and exposure to ionizing radiation.

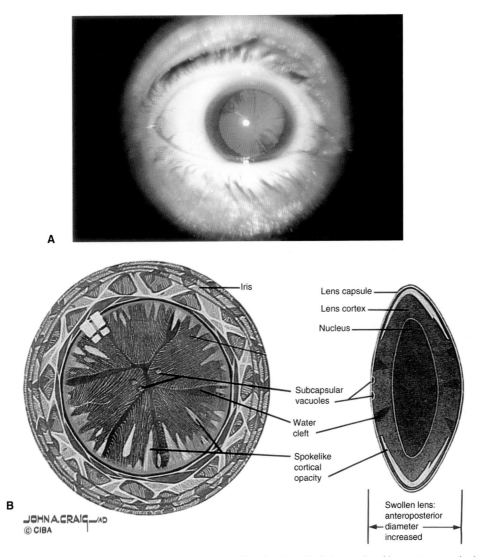

Figure 5-4 **A**, Cortical cataract viewed by retroillumination. **B**, Schematic of immature cortical cataract. *(Courtesy of CIBA Pharmaceutical Co., division of CIBA-GEIGY Corp. Reproduced with permission from* Clinical Symposia. *Illustration by John A. Craig.)*

Histopathologically, PSC is associated with posterior migration of the lens epithelial cells in the posterior subcapsular area, with aberrant enlargement. The swollen epithelial cells are called Wedl, or bladder, cells.

Kuszak JR, Deutsch TA, Brown HG. Anatomy of aged and senile cataractous lenses. In: Albert DM, Jakobiec FA, eds. *Principles and Practice of Ophthalmology.* Philadelphia: Saunders; 1994:564–575.

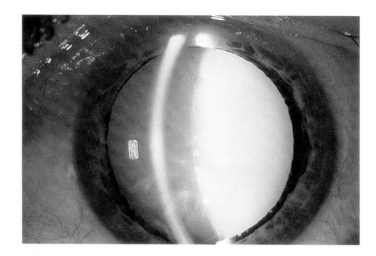

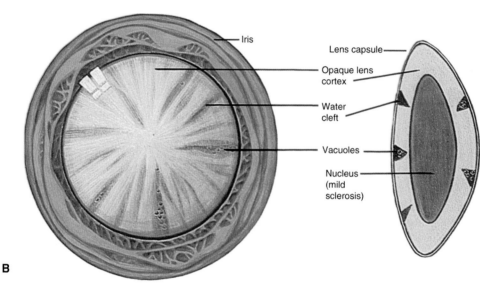

Iris

Lens capsule

Opaque lens
cortex

Water
cleft

Vacuoles

Nucleus
(mild
sclerosis)

Figure 5-5 **A**, Mature cortical cataract. **B**, Schematic of mature cortical cataract. *(Courtesy of CIBA Pharmaceutical Co., division of CIBA-GEIGY Corp. Reproduced with permission from* Clinical Symposia. *Illustration by John A. Craig.)*

Drug-Induced Lens Changes

Corticosteroids

Long-term use of corticosteroids may cause PSCs. Their incidence is related to dose and duration of treatment, and individual susceptibility to corticosteroid-induced PSCs appears to vary. Cataract formation has been reported following administration of corticosteroids by several routes: systemic, topical, subconjunctival, and through nasal sprays.

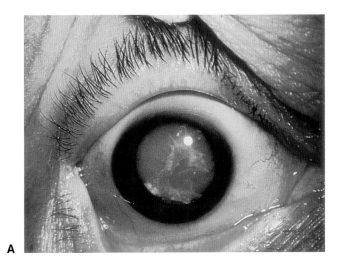

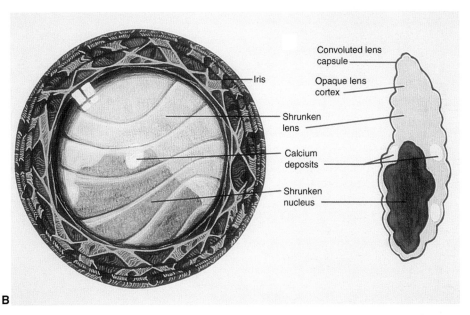

Figure 5-6 **A**, Hypermature cortical cataract. **B**, Schematic of hypermature cortical cataract. *(Courtesy of CIBA Pharmaceutical Co., division of CIBA-GEIGY Corp. Reproduced with permission from* Clinical Symposia. *Illustration by John A. Craig.)*

For example, cataracts have been reported following prolonged treatment of eyelid dermatitis with topical corticosteroids.

In one study of patients treated with oral prednisone and observed for 1–4 years, 11% treated with 10 mg/day of prednisone developed cataracts, as did 30% of those receiving 10–15 mg/day and 80% of those receiving more than 15 mg/day. In another study, half of the patients receiving topical corticosteroids following keratoplasty devel-

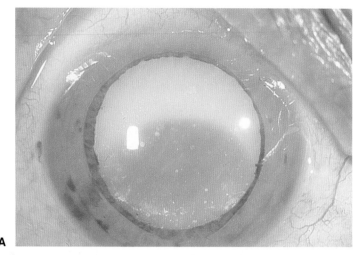

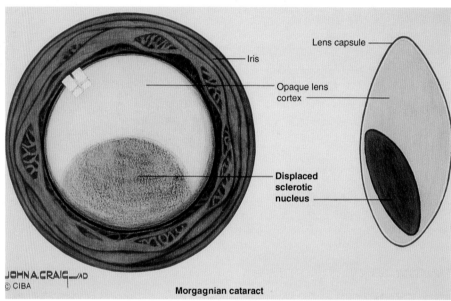

Figure 5-7 A, Morgagnian cataract. **B**, Schematic of morgagnian cataract. *(Courtesy of CIBA Pharmaceutical Co., division of CIBA-GEIGY Corp. Reproduced with permission from Clinical Symposia. Illustration by John A. Craig.)*

oped cataracts after receiving an average of 2.4 drops per day of 0.1% dexamethasone over a period of 10.5 months.

Histopathologically and clinically, PSC formation occurring subsequent to corticosteroid use cannot be distinguished from senescent PSC changes. Some steroid-induced PSCs in children may be reversible with cessation of the drug.

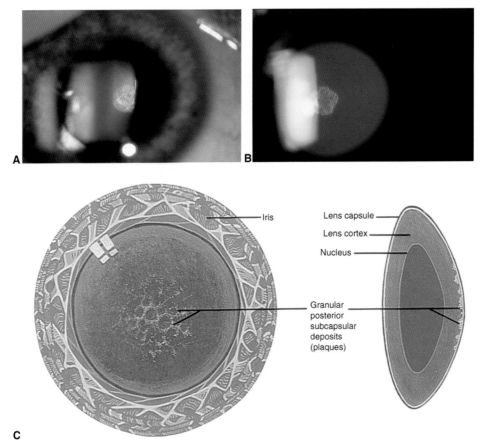

Figure 5-8 Posterior subcapsular cataract (PSC) viewed at the slit lamp **(A)** and with indirect illumination **(B)**. **C**, Schematic of PSC. *(Courtesy of CIBA Pharmaceutical Co., division of CIBA-GEIGY Corp. Reproduced with permission from* Clinical Symposia. *Illustration by John A. Craig.)*

Phenothiazines

Phenothiazines, a major group of psychotropic medications, can cause pigmented deposits in the anterior lens epithelium in an axial configuration (Fig 5-9). These deposits appear to be dependent on both dose and duration. In addition, they are more likely to be seen with some phenothiazines, notably chlorpromazine and thioridazine, than with others. The visual changes associated with phenothiazine use are generally insignificant.

Miotics

Anticholinesterases can cause cataracts. The incidence of cataracts has been reported as high as 20% in patients after 55 months of pilocarpine use and 60% in patients after phospholine iodide use. Usually, these cataracts first appear as small vacuoles within and posterior to the anterior lens capsule and epithelium. These vacuoles are best appreciated by retroillumination. The cataract may progress to posterior cortical and nuclear lens changes as well. Cataract formation is more likely in patients receiving anticholinesterase

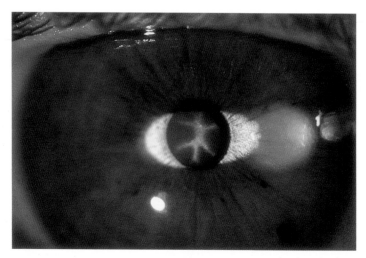

Figure 5-9 Pigmented deposits on anterior lens capsule in patient treated with phenothiazines.

therapy over a long period of time and in those receiving more frequent dosage. Although visually significant cataracts are common in elderly patients receiving topical anticholinesterases, progressive cataract formation has not been reported in children treated with echothiophate for accommodative esotropia.

Amiodarone

Amiodarone, an antiarrhythmia medication, has been reported to cause stellate anterior axial pigment deposition. Only very rarely is this condition visually significant. Amiodarone is also deposited in the corneal epithelium and rarely causes optic neuropathy.

Statins

Studies in dogs have shown that some 3-hydroxy-3-methylglutaryl coenzyme A (HMG-CoA) reductase inhibitors (statins) are associated with cataract when administered in excessive doses. Long-term use of statins in humans has been shown to not be associated with an increased cataract risk. However, concomitant use of simvastatin and erythromycin may be associated with an approximately two- to threefold increased risk of cataract.

Schlienger RG, Haefeli WE, Jick H, et al. Risk of cataract in patients treated with statins. *Arch Intern Med.* 2001;161:2021–2026.

Trauma

Traumatic lens damage may be caused by mechanical injury, physical forces (radiation, electrical current, chemicals), and osmotic influences (diabetes mellitus).

Contusion

Vossius ring

Blunt injury to the eye can sometimes cause pigment from the pupillary ruff to be imprinted onto the anterior surface of the lens in a Vossius ring. Although a Vossius ring is visually insignificant and gradually resolves with time, it serves as an indicator of prior blunt trauma.

Traumatic cataract

A blunt, nonperforating injury may cause lens opacification either as an acute event or as a late sequela. A contusion cataract may involve only a portion of the lens or the entire lens. Often, the initial manifestation of a contusion cataract is a stellate or rosette-shaped opacification, usually axial in location, that involves the posterior lens capsule (Fig 5-10). This *rosette cataract* may progress to opacification of the entire lens. In some cases, blunt trauma causes both dislocation and cataract formation (Fig 5-11). Mild contusion cataracts can improve spontaneously in rare cases.

Dislocation and subluxation

During a blunt injury to the eye, rapid expansion of the globe in an equatorial plane can follow compression. This rapid equatorial expansion can disrupt the zonular fibers, causing dislocation or subluxation of the lens. The lens may be dislocated in any direction, including posteriorly into the vitreous cavity or anteriorly into the anterior chamber.

Symptoms and signs of traumatic lens subluxation include fluctuation of vision, impaired accommodation, monocular diplopia, and high astigmatism. Often, iridodonesis or phacodonesis is present. Retroillumination of the lens at the slit lamp through a dilated pupil may reveal the zonular disruption. In some cases, blunt trauma causes both dislocation and cataract formation.

Perforating and Penetrating Injury

A perforating or penetrating injury of the lens often results in opacification of the cortex at the site of the rupture, usually progressing rapidly to complete opacification (Fig 5-12). Occasionally, a small perforating injury of the lens capsule may heal, resulting in a stationary focal cortical cataract (Fig 5-13).

Radiation-Induced Cataracts

Ionizing radiation

The lens is extremely sensitive to ionizing radiation; however, as much as 20 years may pass after exposure before a cataract becomes clinically apparent. This period of latency is related to the dose of radiation and to the patient's age; younger patients are more susceptible because they have more actively growing lens cells. Ionizing radiation in the x-ray range (0.001–10.0 nm wavelength) can cause cataracts in some individuals in dosages as low as 200 rads in one fraction. (A routine chest x-ray equals 0.1 rad exposure to the thorax.)

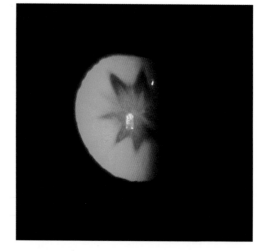

Figure 5-10 Stellate lens opacity following contusion.

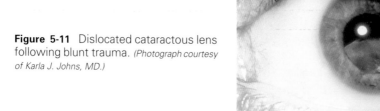

Figure 5-11 Dislocated cataractous lens following blunt trauma. *(Photograph courtesy of Karla J. Johns, MD.)*

The first clinical signs of radiation-induced cataract are often punctate opacities within the posterior capsule and feathery anterior subcapsular opacities that radiate toward the equator of the lens. These opacities may progress to complete opacification of the lens.

Infrared radiation (glassblowers' cataract)

Exposure of the eye to infrared radiation and intense heat over time can cause the outer layers of the anterior lens capsule to peel off as a single layer. Such true exfoliation of the lens capsule, in which the exfoliated outer lamella tends to scroll up on itself, is rarely seen today. Cortical cataract may be associated. (See the section Exfoliation Syndromes.)

Ultraviolet radiation

Experimental evidence suggests that the lens is susceptible to damage from ultraviolet radiation in the UV-B range of 290–320 nm. Epidemiologic evidence and population-based studies indicate that long-term exposure to even low levels of UV-B from sun

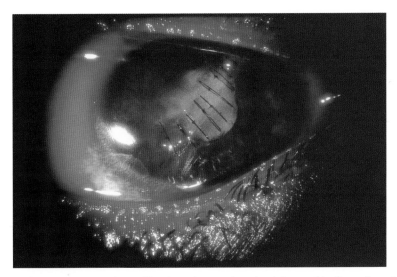

Figure 5-12 Complete cortical opacification after perforating injury, with disruption of the lens capsule.

exposure is associated with an increased risk of cortical and posterior subcapsular cataracts. Ultraviolet-absorbing corrective lenses and nonprescription sunglasses decrease UV transmission by more than 80%, and wearing a hat with a brim decreases ocular sun exposure by 30%–50%.

Microwave radiation

Microwave radiation has been shown to cause cataracts in laboratory animals. Human case reports and epidemiologic studies are more controversial and less conclusive than experimental studies. Cataracts caused by microwave radiation are likely to be anterior and/or posterior subcapsular opacities.

Chemical Injuries

Alkali injuries to the ocular surface often result in cataract, in addition to damaging the cornea, conjunctiva, and iris. Alkali compounds penetrate the eye readily, causing an increase in aqueous pH and a decrease in the level of aqueous glucose and ascorbate. Cortical cataract formation may occur acutely or as a delayed effect of chemical injury. Because acid tends to penetrate the eye less easily than alkali, acid injuries are less likely to result in cataract formation.

Intralenticular Foreign Bodies

Rarely, a small foreign body can perforate the cornea and the anterior lens capsule and become lodged within the lens. If the foreign body is not composed of a ferric or cupric material, and the anterior lens capsule seals the perforation site, the foreign body may be retained within the lens without significant complication. Intralenticular foreign bodies may cause cataract formation in some cases but do not always lead to lens opacification.

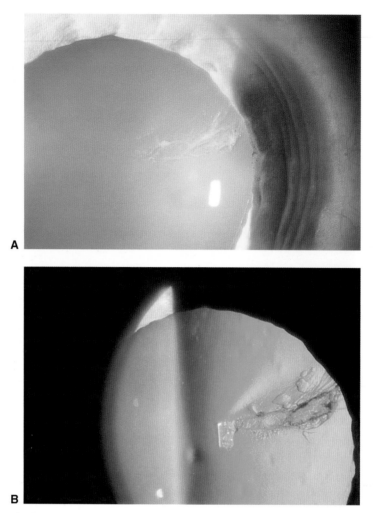

Figure 5-13 A, Focal cortical cataract from a small perforating injury to the lens capsule. **B**, Focal cortical cataract viewed by retroillumination.

Metallosis

Siderosis bulbi

Iron intraocular foreign bodies can result in siderosis bulbi, a condition characterized by deposition of iron molecules in the trabecular meshwork, lens epithelium, iris, and retina (Fig 5-14A). The epithelium and cortical fibers of the affected lens at first show a yellowish tinge, followed later by a rusty brown discoloration (Fig 5-14B). Lens involvement occurs more rapidly if the retained foreign body is embedded close to the lens. Later manifestations of siderosis bulbi are complete cortical cataract formation and retinal dysfunction.

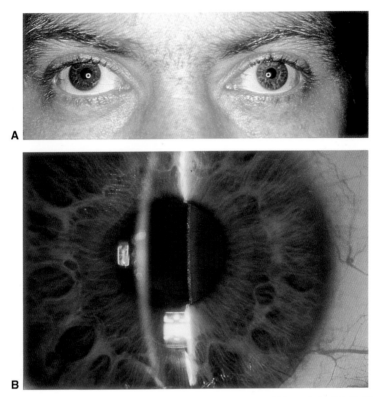

Figure 5-14 Siderosis bulbi. **A**, Heterochromia iridis caused by siderosis bulbi. **B**, Discoloration of lens capsule and cortex.

Chalcosis

Chalcosis occurs when an intraocular copper-containing foreign body deposits copper in Descemet's membrane, the anterior lens capsule, and other intraocular basement membranes. A *sunflower cataract* is a petal-shaped deposition of yellow or brown pigmentation in the lens capsule that radiates from the anterior axial pole of the lens to its equator. Usually, the sunflower cataract causes no significant loss of visual acuity. However, intraocular foreign bodies containing almost pure copper (more than 90%) can cause a severe inflammatory reaction and intraocular necrosis.

Electrical Injury

Electrical shock can cause protein coagulation and cataract formation. Lens manifestations are more likely when the transmission of current involves the patient's head. Initially, lens vacuoles appear in the anterior midperiphery of the lens, followed by linear opacities in the anterior subcapsular cortex. Cataracts induced by electrical injuries may regress, remain stationary, or mature to complete cataract over months or years (Fig 5-15).

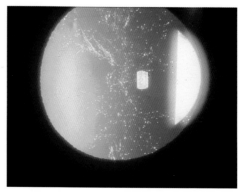

Figure 5-15 Electrical injury. *(Photograph courtesy of Karla J. Johns, MD.)*

Portellos M, Orlin SE, Kozart DM. Electric cataracts [photo essay]. *Arch Ophthalmol.* 1996;114:1022–1023.

Metabolic Cataract

Diabetes Mellitus

Diabetes mellitus can affect the clarity of the lens, its refractive index, and its accommodative amplitude. As the blood sugar level increases, so also does the glucose content in the aqueous humor. Because glucose from the aqueous enters the lens by diffusion, glucose content in the lens will likewise be increased. Some of the glucose is converted by the enzyme aldose reductase to sorbitol, which is not metabolized but remains in the lens.

Subsequently, osmotic pressure causes an influx of water into the lens, which leads to swelling of the lens fibers. The state of lenticular hydration can affect the refractive power of the lens. Patients with diabetes may show transient refractive changes owing to changes in their blood sugar. Acute myopic shifts may indicate undiagnosed or poorly controlled diabetes. People with diabetes have a decreased amplitude of accommodation compared to age-matched controls, and presbyopia may present at a younger age in patients with diabetes than in those without.

Cataract is a common cause of visual impairment in patients with diabetes. Although 2 types of cataract are classically observed in these patients, other patterns may also be encountered. The true *diabetic cataract*, or *snowflake cataract*, consists of bilateral, widespread subcapsular lens changes of abrupt onset and acute progression, typically in young people with uncontrolled diabetes mellitus (Fig 5-16). Multiple gray-white subcapsular opacities that have a snowflake appearance are seen initially in the superficial anterior and posterior lens cortex. Vacuoles appear in the lens capsule, and clefts form in the underlying cortex. Intumescence and maturity of the cortical cataract follow shortly thereafter. Researchers believe that the underlying metabolic changes associated with the true diabetic cataract in humans are closely allied to the sorbitol cataract studied in experimental animals. Although true diabetic cataracts are rarely encountered in clinical

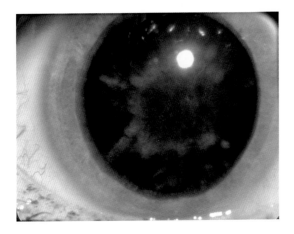

Figure 5-16 Diabetic cataract, also called snowflake cataract, consists of gray-white subcapsular opacities. This type of cataract is seen, in rare cases, in patients with uncontrolled diabetes mellitus. *(Photograph courtesy of Karla J. Johns, MD.)*

practice today, any rapidly maturing bilateral cortical cataracts in a child or young adult should alert the clinician to the possibility of diabetes mellitus.

The *senescent cataract* is the second type frequently observed in patients with diabetes. Evidence suggests that these patients have increased risk of age-related lens changes indistinguishable from nondiabetic age-related cataracts, and that these lens changes tend to occur at a younger age than in patients without diabetes. The high risk of age-related cataracts in patients with diabetes may be a result of the accumulation of sorbitol within the lens, subsequent hydration changes, and the increased glycosylation of proteins in the diabetic lens.

Flynn HW, Jr, Smiddy WE, eds. *Diabetes and Ocular Disease: Past, Present, and Future Therapies.* Ophthalmology Monograph 14. San Francisco: American Academy of Ophthalmology; 2000:49–53, 226.

Galactosemia

Galactosemia is an inherited autosomal recessive inability to convert galactose to glucose. As a consequence of this inability, excessive galactose accumulates in body tissues, with further metabolic conversion of galactose to galactitol (dulcitol), the sugar alcohol of galactose. Galactosemia can result from defects in 1 of 3 enzymes involved in the metabolism of galactose: galactose–1-phosphate uridyl transferase, galactokinase, or UDP-galactose-4-epimerase. The most common and the severest form, known as classic galactosemia, is caused by a defect in the enzyme transferase.

In *classic galactosemia,* symptoms of malnutrition, hepatomegaly, jaundice, and mental deficiency present within the first few weeks of life. The disease is fatal if undiagnosed and untreated. The diagnosis of classic galactosemia can be confirmed by demonstration of the non–glucose-reducing substance galactose in the urine.

Of patients with classic galactosemia, 75% will develop cataract, usually within the first few weeks after birth. Accumulation of galactose and galactitol within the lens cells leads to increased intracellular osmotic pressure and fluid influx into the lens. Typically, the nucleus and deep cortex become increasingly opacified, causing an "oil droplet" appearance on retroillumination (Fig 5-17). If the disease remains untreated, the cataracts

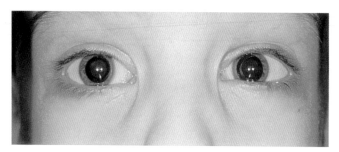

Figure 5-17 "Oil droplet" bilateral cataracts in galactosemia.

progress to total opacification of the lens. Treatment of galactosemia includes elimination of milk and milk products from the diet. In some cases, early cataract formation can be reversed by timely diagnosis and dietary intervention.

Deficiencies of the 2 other enzymes, galactokinase and epimerase, can also cause galactosemia. These deficiencies are less common, however, and cause less severe systemic abnormalities. Cataracts caused by deficiencies in these enzymes may be seen, but they tend to present later in life than those seen in classic galactosemia.

Hypocalcemia (Tetanic Cataract)

Cataracts may occur in association with any condition that results in hypocalcemia. *Hypocalcemia* may be idiopathic, or it may appear as a result of unintended destruction of the parathyroid glands during thyroid surgery. Usually bilateral, hypocalcemic cataracts are punctate iridescent opacities in the anterior and posterior cortex that lie beneath the lens capsule and are usually separated from it by a zone of clear lens. These discrete opacities may either remain stable or mature into complete cortical cataracts.

Wilson Disease (Hepatolenticular Degeneration)

Wilson disease is an inherited autosomal recessive disorder of copper metabolism. The characteristic ocular manifestation of Wilson disease is the Kayser-Fleischer ring, a golden brown discoloration of Descemet's membrane around the periphery of the cornea. In addition, a characteristic sunflower cataract often develops. Reddish brown pigment (cuprous oxide) is deposited in the anterior lens capsule and subcapsular cortex in a stellate shape that resembles the petals of a sunflower. In most cases, the sunflower cataract does not produce serious visual impairment.

Myotonic Dystrophy

Myotonic dystrophy is an inherited autosomal dominant condition characterized by delayed relaxation of contracted muscles, ptosis, weakness of the facial musculature, cardiac conduction defects, and prominent frontal balding in affected male patients. Patients with this disorder typically develop polychromatic iridescent crystals in the lens cortex (Fig 5-18), with sequential PSC progressing to complete cortical opacification. Ultrastructurally, these crystals are composed of whorls of plasmalemma from the lens fibers. Subsequently, there is PSC formation and opacification of the lens cortex. Iridescent

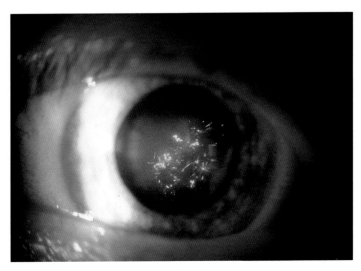

Figure 5-18 Myotonic dystrophy. *(Photograph courtesy of Karla J. Johns, MD.)*

polychromatic crystals are occasionally seen in the lens cortex of patients who do not have myotonic dystrophy and are thought to be caused by cholesterol crystal deposition in the lens.

Nutritional Effects

Although nutritional deficiencies have been demonstrated to cause cataracts in animal models, this etiology has been difficult to confirm in humans. Epidemiologic evidence published over the past decade has conflicting information on this subject. Some studies have suggested that multivitamins, vitamin A, vitamin C, vitamin E, niacin, thiamine, riboflavin, beta carotene, and increased protein may have a protective effect on cataract development. Other studies have found that vitamins C and E have little or no effect on cataract development. Most recently, the Age-Related Eye Disease Study (AREDS) showed that over 7 years, increased intake of vitamins C and E and beta carotene did not decrease the development or progression of cataract. However, high-dosage vitamin use does carry risk. Smokers taking high doses of vitamin A and beta carotene have been shown to have an increased risk of lung cancer, of death from lung cancer, and of death from cardio-vascular disease.

Lutein and zeaxanthin are the only carotenoids found in human lenses, and recent studies have shown a moderate decrease in the risk of cataract with the increased frequency of intake of food high in lutein (spinach, kale, and broccoli). Eating cooked spinach more than twice a week decreased the risk of cataract. This decreased risk was unrelated to healthy lifestyle. In contrast to the effects of such dietary supplements, severe episodes of diarrhea associated with severe dehydration may be associated with increased risk of cataract formation.

Prospective studies of men and women have determined that cigarette smoking increases the risk of PSCs and nuclear sclerosis in both sexes.

Age-Related Eye Disease Study Research Group. A randomized, placebo-controlled, clinical trial of high-dose supplementation with vitamins C and E and beta carotene for age-related cataract and vision loss: AREDS report no. 9. *Arch Ophthalmol.* 2001;119:1439–1452.

Berendschot TT, Broekmans WM, Klopping-Ketalaars IA, et al. Lens aging in relation to nutritional determinants and possible risk factors for age-related cataract. *Arch Ophthalmol.* 2002;120:1732–1737.

Chasan-Taber L, Willett WC, Seddon JM, et al. A prospective study of carotenoid and vitamin A intakes and risk of cataract extraction in US women. *Am J Clin Nutr.* 1999;70:509–516.

Christen WG, Manson JE, Seddon JM, et al. A prospective study of cigarette smoking and risk of cataract in men. *JAMA.* 1992;268:989–993.

Cumming RG, Mitchell P, Smith W. Diet and cataract: the Blue Mountains Eye Study. *Ophthalmology.* 2000;107:450–456.

Hankinson SE, Willett WC, Colditz GA, et al. A prospective study of cigarette smoking and risk of cataract surgery in women. *JAMA.* 1992;268:994–998.

Leske MC, Chylack LT Jr, He Q, et al. Antioxidant vitamins and nuclear opacities: the longitudinal study of cataract. *Ophthalmology.* 1998;105:831–836.

Lyle BJ, Mares-Perlman JA, Klein BE, et al. Antioxidant intake and risk of incident age-related nuclear cataracts in the Beaver Dam Eye Study. *Am J Epidemiol.* 1999;149:801–809.

Omenn GS, Goodman GE, Thornquist MD, et al. Effects of a combination of beta carotene and vitamin A on lung cancer and cardiovascular disease. *N Engl J Med.* 1996;334:1150–1155.

Cataract Associated With Uveitis

Lens changes often occur secondary to chronic uveitis and/or associated corticosteroid therapy. Typically, a PSC appears; anterior lens changes may also occur (Fig 5-19). The formation of posterior synechiae is common in uveitis, often with thickening of the anterior lens capsule, which may have an associated fibrous pupillary membrane. Lens changes in cataract secondary to uveitis may progress to a mature cataract. Calcium deposits may be observed on the anterior capsule or within the lens substance.

Cortical cataract formation occurs in up to 70% of cases of Fuchs heterochromic uveitis (see Fig 5-19). Because posterior synechiae do not commonly occur in this syndrome, formation of pupillary membranes is unlikely and chronic corticosteroid therapy is not indicated. Cataract extraction in patients with Fuchs heterochromic uveitis generally has a favorable prognosis. Intraoperative anterior chamber hemorrhages have been reported in approximately 25% of cases.

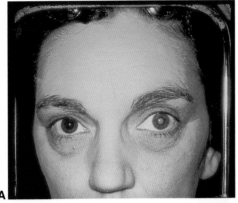

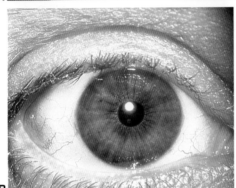

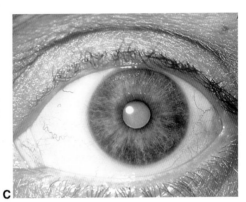

Figure 5-19 Fuchs heterochromic uveitis. **A**, Patient with Fuchs heterochromic uveitis. In this case, the affected eye is lighter. **B**, Normal right eye. **C**, Cataract formation in affected left eye. *(Photographs courtesy of Karla J. Johns, MD.)*

Exfoliation Syndromes

True Exfoliation

True exfoliation of the lens capsule is rare, occurring primarily in glassblowers and blast furnace operators. Presumably, intense exposure to infrared radiation and heat causes the superficial lens capsule to delaminate and peel off in scrolls.

Exfoliation Syndrome (Pseudoexfoliation)

In *exfoliation syndrome,* a basement membrane–like fibrillogranular white material is deposited on the lens, cornea, iris, anterior hyaloid face, ciliary processes, zonular fibers, and trabecular meshwork. These deposits, believed to arise from basement membranes within the eye, appear as grayish white flecks that are prominent at the pupillary margin and on the lens capsule (Fig 5-20). Associated with this condition are atrophy of the iris at the pupillary margin, deposition of pigment on the anterior surface of the iris, poorly dilating pupil, increased pigmentation of the trabecular meshwork, capsular fragility, zonular weakness, and open-angle glaucoma. Exfoliation syndrome is a unilateral or bilateral disorder that becomes more apparent with increasing age.

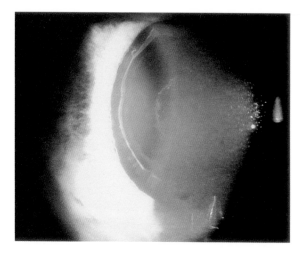

Figure 5-20 Exfoliation syndrome (pseudoexfoliation).

Some investigators have reported an increased prevalence of senescent cataracts in patients with exfoliation syndrome. Patients with this syndrome may also experience weakness of the zonular fibers and spontaneous lens subluxation and phacodonesis. Poor zonular integrity may affect cataract surgery technique and IOL implantation. The exfoliative material may be elaborated even after the crystalline lens is removed.

Naumann GO, Schlotzer-Schrehardt U, Kuchle M. Pseudoexfoliation syndrome for the comprehensive ophthalmologist. Intraocular and systemic manifestations. *Ophthalmology.* 1998;105:951–968.

Ritch R. Exfoliation syndrome. *Focal Points: Clinical Modules for Ophthalmologists.* San Francisco: American Academy of Ophthalmology; 1994, module 9.

Cataract and Skin Diseases

Atopic Dermatitis

Atopic dermatitis is a chronic, itching, erythematous dermatitis, often seen in conjunction with increased levels of immunoglobulin E (IgE) and a history of multiple allergies or asthma. Cataract formation has been reported in up to 25% of patients with atopic dermatitis. The cataracts are usually bilateral, and onset occurs in the second to third decade. Typically, these cataracts are anterior subcapsular opacities in the pupillary area that resemble shieldlike plaques.

Mannis MJ, Macsai MS, Huntley AC, eds. *Eye and Skin Disease.* Philadelphia: Lippincott-Raven; 1996.

Lens-Induced Uveitis

Phacoantigenic Uveitis (Phacoanaphylactic Uveitis)

In the normal eye, minute amounts of lens proteins leak out through the lens capsule. The eye appears to have immunologic tolerance to these small amounts of lens antigens. However, the liberation of a large amount of lens protein into the anterior chamber disrupts this immunologic tolerance and may trigger a severe inflammatory reaction. *Phacoantigenic uveitis*, sometimes referred to as *phacoanaphylactic uveitis*, is an immune-mediated granulomatous inflammation initiated by lens proteins released through a ruptured lens capsule. Phacoantigenic uveitis usually occurs following traumatic rupture of the lens capsule or following cataract surgery when cortical material is retained within the eye. Onset is days to weeks after the injury or surgery.

The disease is characterized by a red, painful eye with chemosis and anterior chamber inflammation with cells, flare, and keratic precipitates. Occasionally, glaucoma secondary to blockage of the trabecular meshwork and synechiae formation may occur. Late complications include cyclitic membrane, hypotony, and phthisis bulbi. Rarely, phacoantigenic uveitis can give rise to an inflammatory reaction in the fellow eye. Lens extraction is the definitive therapy for the condition. Histopathologic examination shows a zonal granulomatous inflammation surrounding a breach of the lens capsule. (See BCSC Section 4, *Ophthalmic Pathology and Intraocular Tumors*, and BCSC Section 9, *Intraocular Inflammation and Uveitis*.)

Lens-Induced Glaucoma

Phacolytic Glaucoma

Phacolytic glaucoma is a complication of a mature or hypermature cataract. Denatured, liquefied high-molecular-weight lens proteins leak through an intact but permeable lens capsule. An immune response is not elicited; rather, macrophages ingest these lens proteins. The trabecular meshwork can become clogged with both the lens proteins and the engorged macrophages. The usual clinical presentation of phacolytic glaucoma shows abrupt onset of pain and redness in a cataractous eye that has had poor vision for some time. The cornea may be edematous, and significant flare reaction occurs in the anterior chamber. White flocculent material appears in the anterior chamber and often adheres to the lens capsule as well. Intraocular pressure (IOP) is markedly elevated, and the anterior chamber angle is open, although it may show precipitates of white flocculent material. Initial treatment of phacolytic glaucoma consists of control of the IOP with antiglaucoma medications and of the inflammation with topical corticosteroids. Surgical removal of the lens is the definitive treatment.

Lens-Particle Glaucoma

Following a penetrating lens injury, extracapsular cataract extraction (ECCE) with retained cortical material, or, rarely, Nd:YAG capsulotomy, lens cortex may be liberated into the anterior chamber. Here, it causes an obstruction of aqueous outflow through the trabecular meshwork. In most instances, the onset of glaucoma is delayed by days or weeks after the surgical event or lens injury. Examination reveals white, fluffy, cortical lens material in the anterior chamber, sometimes in association with an anterior segment inflammatory reaction. Gonioscopy shows that the angle is open, and cortical material can often be seen deposited along the trabecular meshwork. Medical therapy to lower IOP and to reduce intraocular inflammation is indicated. If the IOP and inflammation do not respond quickly to this treatment, surgical removal of the retained lens material may be required.

Phacomorphic Glaucoma

An intumescent cataractous lens can cause pupillary block and induce secondary angle-closure glaucoma, or it can physically push the iris forward and thus cause shallowing of the anterior chamber. Typically, the patient presents with a red, painful eye and a history of decreased vision as a result of cataract formation prior to the acute event (Fig 5-21). The cornea may be edematous. The anterior chamber is shallow, and gonioscopy reveals a closed anterior chamber angle. Initial management includes medical treatment to lower IOP. The condition responds to laser iridotomy, but definitive treatment consists of cataract extraction.

Glaukomflecken

Glaukomflecken are gray-white epithelial and anterior cortical lens opacities that occur following an episode of markedly elevated IOP, as in acute angle-closure glaucoma. Histopathologically, glaukomflecken are composed of necrotic lens epithelial cells and degenerated subepithelial cortex.

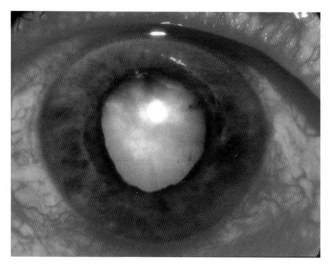

Figure 5-21 Phacomorphic glaucoma.

Ischemia

Ischemic ocular conditions, such as pulseless disease (Takayasu arteritis), thromboangiitis obliterans (Buerger disease), and anterior segment necrosis, can cause PSC. The cataract may progress rapidly to total opacification of the lens.

Cataracts Associated With Degenerative Ocular Disorders

Cataracts can occur secondary to many degenerative ocular diseases, such as retinitis pigmentosa, essential iris atrophy, chronic hypotony, and absolute glaucoma. These secondary cataracts usually begin as PSCs and may progress to total lens opacification. There are various mechanisms of cataractogenesis in degenerative ocular disorders.

Burke JP, O'Keefe M, Bowell R, et al. Ophthalmic findings in classical galactosemia: a screened population. *J Pediatr Ophthalmol Strabismus.* 1989;26:165–168.

Cruickshanks KF, Klein BE, Klein R. Ultraviolet light exposure and lens opacities: the Beaver Dam Eye Study. *Am J Public Health.* 1992;82:1658–1662.

Edwards MC, Johnson JL, Marriage B, et al. Isolated sulfite oxidase deficiency: review of two cases in one family. *Ophthalmology.* 1999;106:1957–1961.

Fraunfelder FT, Fraunfelder FW. *Drug-Induced Ocular Side Effects.* 5th ed. Boston: Butterworth-Heinemann; 2001.

Gold DH, Weingeist TA, eds. *The Eye in Systemic Disease.* Philadelphia: Lippincott; 1990:90, 330–331, 390, 434.

Havener WH. *Ocular Pharmacology.* 5th ed. St Louis: Mosby; 1983:366, 487–489.

Irvine JA, Smith RE. Lens injuries. In: Shingleton BJ, Hersh PS, Kenyon KR, eds. *Eye Trauma.* St Louis: Mosby; 1991:126–135.

Johns KJ. Diabetes and the lens. In: Feman SS, ed. *Ocular Problems in Diabetes Mellitus.* Boston: Blackwell; 1992:221–244.

Klein BE, Klein R, Lee KE. Incidence of age-related cataract: the Beaver Dam Eye Study. *Arch Ophthalmol.* 1998;116:219–225.

Liebman JM, Ritch R. Glaucoma secondary to lens intumescence and dislocation. In: Ritch R, Shields MB, Krupin T, eds. *The Glaucomas.* 2nd ed. St Louis: Mosby; 1996.

Lipman RM, Tripathi BJ, Tripathi RC. Cataracts induced by microwave and ionizing radiation. *Surv Ophthalmol.* 1988;33:200–210.

Nelson LB, Spaeth GL, Nowinski TS, et al. Aniridia: a review. *Surv Ophthalmol.* 1984;28:621–642.

Richter C, Epstein DL. Lens-induced open-angle glaucoma. In: Ritch R, Shields MB, Krupin T, eds. *The Glaucomas.* 2nd ed. St Louis: Mosby; 1996.

Urban RC Jr, Cotlier E. Corticosteroid-induced cataracts. *Surv Ophthalmol.* 1986;31:102–110.

West SK, Duncan DD, Muñoz B, et al. Sunlight exposure and risk of lens opacities in a population-based study: the Salisbury Eye Evaluation Project. *JAMA.* 1998;280:714–718.

West SK, Valmadrid CT. Epidemiology of risk factors for age-related cataract. *Surv Ophthalmol.* 1995;39:323–334.

Young RW. *Age-Related Cataract.* New York: Oxford University Press; 1991.

CHAPTER 6

Epidemiology of Cataracts

According to the World Health Organization (WHO), cataract is the leading cause of blindness and visual impairment throughout the world. With the general aging of the population, the overall prevalence of visual loss as a result of lenticular opacities increases each year. Cataracts cause reversible blindness in more than 17 million people worldwide, and this figure is projected to reach 40 million by year 2020. The WHO projects that between 2000 and 2020 the number of cataract surgeries performed worldwide will need to triple. Currently in the United States, more than 5000 cataract surgeries/million population are performed, whereas in China, the number is fewer than 500 cataract surgeries/million population. It has been shown that visual impairment and age-related cataract may be independent risk factors for increased mortality in older persons. Cataract affects nearly 20.5 million Americans age 40 and older, or about 1 in every 6 people in this age range. About 1.6 million cataract procedures were performed on Medicare beneficiaries in 2000.

Because surgery is the only treatment currently available for visually significant lenticular opacity, the growing need for surgical resources compounds the already significant socioeconomic impact of cataracts in particular and blindness in general. The problem is especially critical in developing countries, where 1 blind individual takes 2 individuals out of the work force, if the blind person requires the care of an able adult.

The economic impact of cataract surgery in the United States alone is enormous. It is estimated that the federal government spends more than $3.4 billion each year treating cataract through the Medicare program. In addition to the vast number of cataract operations performed each year in the United States, an even greater number of related office visits and tests contribute to the financial impact of cataract surgery.

Although cataracts may be congenital, metabolic, or traumatic in origin, senile cataracts have the greatest socioeconomic impact because of their prevalence. The lack of a widely accepted standardized classification system for lens opacities makes it difficult to evaluate precisely the prevalence and incidence of cataracts. The size, shape, density, and location of age-related lens opacities are variable, and most definitions of cataract require a quantifiable reduction in visual acuity in addition to alterations in lens morphology visible at the slit lamp. Further, examination methods are often subjective and require patient participation, and thus studies are easily biased. Most estimates of senile cataract frequency are based on data from selective groups rather than from general populations. Finally, in many elderly patients, eyes may have a coexisting pathology, producing visual loss that might have been incorrectly attributed to lens changes.

A number of studies on cataract have been carried out in recent years. The Age-Related Eye Disease Study (AREDS) was performed during the 1990s. Among other findings, the study demonstrated a high degree of reliability in grading the severity of lens opacities in a large study cohort with mostly early lens changes. The AREDS system for classifying cataracts from photography may be useful in future studies of cataract incidence and progression.

Age-Related Eye Disease Study Research Group. The age-related eye disease study (AREDS) system for classifying cataracts from photographs: AREDS report no. 4. *Am J Ophthalmol.* 2001;131:167–175.

The Beaver Dam Eye Study was a large population-based study that was performed in the late 1980s (data published in the 1990s). It reported that 38.8% of men and 45.9% of women older than 74 years had visually significant cataracts. For this study, "significance" was determined by photographic grading of lens opacities and best-corrected visual acuity of 20/32 (logMAR equivalent closest to 20/30 Snellen fraction), excluding those with severe age-related maculopathy. The incidence of cataract in this study is shown in Table 6-1.

A follow-up to the Beaver Dam Eye Study was performed between 1993 and 1995 to estimate the incidence of nuclear, cortical, and posterior subcapsular cataract (PSC) in the study cohort. Incident nuclear cataract occurred in 13.1%, cortical cataract in 8.2%, and PSC in 3.4%. The cumulative incidence of nuclear cataract increased from 2.9% in ages 43–54 years at baseline to 40.0% in those ages 75 years or older. For cortical and PSC, the corresponding values were 1.9% and 21.8% and 1.4% and 7.3%, respectively. Women were more likely than men to have nuclear cataracts, even after adjusting for age.

Klein BE, Klein R, Lee KE. Incidence of age-related cataract: the Beaver Eye Study. *Arch Ophthalmol.* 1998;116:219–225.

The Baltimore Eye Survey revealed that cataract was the leading cause of blindness (20/200 or worse vision) among those 40 years and older. Untreated cataract was the source of blindness in 27% of African Americans and 13% of Caucasians.

Table 6-1 Percent Prevalence of Visually Significant* Cataract in the Beaver Dam Eye Study, 1988–1990

Age	Women		Men	
	Worse Eye (%)	Better Eye (%)	Worse Eye (%)	Better Eye (%)
43–54	2.6	0.4	0.4	0.0
55–64	10.0	1.0	3.9	0.3
65–74	23.5	8.3	14.3	3.4
75+	45.9	25.4	38.8	12.6

* Visually significant indicates visual acuity in the affected eye of 20/32 or worse (Snellen fraction equivalent of 45 letters correct on logMAR chart). This excludes subjects with geographic atrophy or exudative maculopathy in the affected eye.

(Adapted from Klein BK, Klein R, Linton KL. Prevalence of age-related lens opacities in a population. The Beaver Dam Eye Study. *Ophthalmology.* 1992;99:546–552.)

The Longitudinal Study of Cataract (LSC) was an epidemiologic study of the natural history of and risk factors for lens opacities. In this study, nuclear opacification was linked with increasing age, white race, lower education, gout medication, current smoking, family history of cataract, preexisting PSC, and early use of eye glasses. The LSC assessed new lens opacities and the progression of lenticular opacities using a research instrument called the *Lens Opacities Classification System III (LOCS III)*. The median age of study participants was 65 years, and the incidence of new opacities was 6% after 2 years and 8% after 5 years. After 5 years' follow-up, the incidence rates for developing cortical and posterior subcapsular opacities were 7.7% and 4.3%, respectively. Stated another way, after 5 years, 1 in 13 participants developed a new cortical opacity and 1 in 24 developed a new posterior subcapsular opacity. The progression rate of preexisting cortical opacities was 16.2% after 5 years. The progression of preexisting posterior subcapsular opacities was higher, reaching 55.1% after 5 years of follow-up. Although the incidence rates for both cortical and posterior subcapsular opacities were much higher for those aged 65 years or older than for those younger than 65 years, the progression rates for these 2 age groups were very similar.

Leske MC, Chylack LT Jr, He Q, et al. Incidence and progression of cortical and posterior subcapsular opacities: the Longitudinal Study of Cataract. The LSC Group. *Ophthalmology.* 1997;104:1987–1993.

The Barbados Eye Study provides prevalence data on lens opacities in a predominantly black population. Cortical opacities were the most frequent type of cataract, and women had a higher frequency of opacification.

Leske MC, Connell AM, Wu SY, et al. Distribution of intraocular pressure. The Barbados Eye Study. *Arch Ophthalmol.* 1997;115:1051–1057.

Other studies have linked the risk of developing cortical opacities and PSC with higher body mass index (BMI) at baseline and have shown increased risk with increasing BMI over time.

Hiller R, Podgor MJ, Sperduto RD, et al. A longitudinal study of body mass index and lens opacities. The Framingham Studies. *Ophthalmology.* 1998;105:1244–1250.

The AREDS report no. 5 found that persons with moderate nuclear opacities were more likely to be female, nonwhite, and smokers, and to have large macular drusen. Moderate nuclear opacities were less common in people with higher educational status, history of diabetes [only patients with mild background diabetic retinopathy (BDR) were included in the study], and in those taking nonsteroidal anti-inflammatory drugs. Moderate cortical opacities were associated with dark iris color, large macular drusen, weight gain, higher sunlight exposure, and the use of thyroid hormone; they were less common in people with higher educational status.

Reported risk factors for cataract development are not consistent in all studies. One consistent finding in the literature is that cortical cataracts are more common in blacks. Other consistent findings include a higher incidence of nuclear cataract in women, smokers, and those with less education. Cigarette smokers have repeatedly been shown to have an increased risk of developing nuclear lens opacities. Some smoking-related damage to the lens may be reversible, and smoking cessation reduces the risk of cataract by limiting total dose-related damage to the lens.

Christen WG, Glynn RJ, Ajani UA, et al. Smoking cessation and risk of age-related cataract in men. *JAMA*. 2000;284:713–716.

Chylack LT Jr, Wolfe JK, Singer DM, et al. The Lens Opacities Classification System III. The Longitudinal Study of Cataract Study Group. *Arch Ophthalmol*. 1993;111:831–836.

Hiller R, Sperduto RD, Podgor MJ, et al. Cigarette smoking and the risk of development of lens opacities. The Framingham Studies. *Arch Ophthalmol*. 1997;115:1113–1118.

Klein BE, Klein R, Linton KL. Prevalence of age-related lens opacities in a population. The Beaver Dam Eye Study. *Ophthalmology*. 1992;99:546–552.

Leske MC, Chylack LT Jr, He Q, et al. Risk factors for nuclear opalescence in a longitudinal study. LSC Group. *Am J Epidemiol*. 1998;147:36–41.

Leske MC, Chylack LT Jr, Wu SY, et al. Incidence and progression of nuclear opacities in the Longitudinal Study of Cataract. *Ophthalmology*. 1996;103:705–712.

Leske MC, Sperduto RD. The epidemiology of senile cataracts: a review. *Am J Epidemiol*. 1983;118:152–165.

Risk factors associated with age-related nuclear and cortical cataract: a case control study in the Age-Related Eye Disease Study. AREDS report no. 5. *Ophthalmology*. 2001;108:1400–1408.

Sommer A, Tielsch JM, Katz J, et al. Racial differences in the cause-specific prevalence of blindness in east Baltimore. *N Engl J Med*. 1991;325:1412–1417.

CHAPTER 7

Evaluation and Management of Cataracts in Adults

When an ophthalmologist evaluates a patient for cataract surgery, the primary objectives are to determine whether the lens opacity is the principal reason for the decline in visual function and to assess the extent of visual loss and its effect on the patient's ability to carry out those activities of daily living that are important to his or her quality of life. The following questions may be considered in the evaluation and management of cataract:

- Does the lens opacity correspond to the degree of visual impairment?
- Will lens removal provide sufficient functional improvement to warrant surgery?
- Is the patient sufficiently healthy to tolerate surgery?
- Is the patient or another responsible person capable of participating in postoperative care?
- Is the lens opacity secondary to a systemic or ocular condition that must be taken into consideration when planning surgery?

Because cataract surgery is, in the vast majority of cases, an elective procedure, the ophthalmologist should allow sufficient time to obtain the answers to these questions. The following sections provide an outline that can help accomplish this task. Ultimately, it is important that both patient and physician be satisfied that surgery is in the best interest of the patient.

Clinical History: Signs and Symptoms

Decreased Visual Acuity

Cataract patients are often self-referred. The patient or a relative or friend realizes that the patient is visually impaired, and the patient sees an ophthalmologist. For these individuals, the clinical history is straightforward, and the patient tells the ophthalmologist which activities have been curtailed or abandoned. In other situations, the patient realizes, only after an examination, that his or her level of visual acuity has declined. Still others deny they are having any problem until their limitations are demonstrated or privileges are withdrawn because they are no longer visually eligible.

Different types of cataract may have different effects on visual acuity, depending on incident light, pupil size, and degree of myopia (Table 7-1). The overall effect of the cataract on visual function is probably a more appropriate way to determine visual disability than is Snellen acuity alone.

After a careful history has been obtained, the patient should undergo a complete visual examination, beginning with a careful refraction. The development of nuclear sclerotic cataract may increase the dioptric power of the lens, commonly causing a mild to moderate degree of myopia. Asymmetric development of lens-induced myopia may produce disabling anisometropia. Specific testing of vision under conditions other than those of the refraction lane may simulate the situations in which the patient has difficulty performing important activities of daily living.

Glare

Cataract patients often complain of increased glare sensitivity, which may vary in severity from a decrease in contrast sensitivity in brightly lit environments to disabling glare in the daytime or with oncoming car headlights or similar lighting conditions at night. This complaint is particularly prominent with posterior subcapsular cataracts (PSCs). Glare testing attempts to determine the degree of visual impairment caused by the presence of a light source located in the patient's visual field. Many patients tolerate moderate levels of glare with little difficulty. However, some individuals have significant reduction in visual function in glare situations. It is important to use a consistent, reliable method to determine glare sensitivity and to document the resultant loss of visual acuity. (Often third-party payers require that an insured person's visual acuity decline to a specified level before they will approve cataract surgery; documenting the loss of vision secondary to glare may permit the patient to be rehabilitated and to be reimbursed for surgical expenses.)

Contrast Sensitivity

Contrast sensitivity measures the patient's ability to detect subtle variations in shading by using figures that vary in contrast, luminance, and spatial frequency. Because contrast sensitivity is unaffected by difficulties a patient may have seeing in reduced luminance, it may provide a more comprehensive estimate of the visual resolution of the optics of the eye and may demonstrate a significant loss of visual function not appreciated with Snellen testing. However, it is not a specific indicator of visual loss due to cataract. If a reproducible technique is used to measure contrast sensitivity, it affords another source of documentation of visual impairment.

Rubin GS, Adamsons IA, Stark, WJ. Comparison of acuity, contrast sensitivity, and disability glare before and after cataract surgery. *Arch Ophthalmol.* 1993;111:56–61.

Rubin GS, Bandeen-Roche K, Huang GH, et al. The association of multiple visual impairments with self-reported visual disability: SEE project. *Invest Ophthalmol Vis Sci.* 2001;42:64–72.

Myopic Shift

The development of cataract may increase the dioptric power of the lens, commonly causing a mild to moderate degree of myopia. Hyperopic presbyopic patients find their

Table 7-1 Effect of Cataract on Visual Acuity

	Growth Rate	Glare	Effect on Distance	Effect on Near	Induced Myopia
Cortical	2+	1+	1+	1+	none
Nuclear	1+	1+	2+	none	2+
Posterior subcapsular	3+	3+	1+	3+	none

need for distance glasses diminished as they experience this so-called *second sight.* However, as the optical quality of the lens deteriorates, this temporary advantage is lost. This phenomenon is encountered with nuclear sclerotic cataracts. Asymmetric development of lens-induced myopia may produce intolerable anisometropia, prompting consideration of cataract extraction.

Monocular Diplopia or Polyopia

Occasionally, nuclear changes are localized to the inner layers of the lens nucleus, resulting in multiple refractile areas in the center of the lens. Such areas may best be seen within the red reflex by retinoscopy or direct ophthalmoscopy. This type of cataract occasionally results in monocular diplopia or polyopia, including ghost images and occasionally a true second image. Monocular diplopia can also be related to media opacities or other disorders of the eye (see also BCSC Section 5, *Neuro-Ophthalmology*). The pinhole test is an easy method to rule out other etiologies in many cases.

Medical Management

Several nonsurgical approaches may be temporarily effective in improving visual function in patients with cataracts. For example, careful refraction can improve spectacle correction for distance and near vision. Increased ambient illumination and increased spectacle add are also helpful for reading. Pupillary dilation either pharmacologically or by laser pupilloplasty may improve visual function in patients with small axial cataracts by allowing light to pass through the more peripheral portions of the lens, being careful not to induce elevated IOP in those patients with narrow anatomic angles.

Medical management of cataracts is being aggressively researched. Although progress is being made, no commercially available medication has been proven to delay or reverse cataract formation in humans. Aldose reductase inhibitors, which block the conversion of glucose to sorbitol, have been shown to prevent cataracts in animals with experimentally induced diabetes. Other possible agents under investigation to slow or reverse the growth of cataracts include sorbitol-lowering agents, aspirin, glutathione-raising agents, and antioxidant vitamins C and E.

Congdon NG. Prevention strategies for age related cataract: present limitations and future possibilities. *Br J Ophthalmol.* 2001;85:516–520.

Jacques PF, Chylack LT Jr, Hankinson SE, et al. Long-term nutrient intake and early age-related nuclear lens opacities. *Arch Ophthalmol.* 2001;119:1009–1019.

Kador PF. Overview of the current attempts toward the medical treatment of cataract. *Ophthalmology.* 1983;90:352–364.

Kuzniarz M, Mitchell P, Cumming RG, et al. Use of vitamin supplements and cataract: the Blue Mountains Eye Study. *Am J Ophthalmol.* 2001;132:19–26.

Low Vision Aids for Cataract

Some patients with limited visual function from cataract may be helped by optical aids when surgical management is not appropriate. Handheld monoculars of 2.5×, 2.8×, and 4× facilitate spotting objects at a distance, whereas high-add spectacles, magnifiers, and telescopic loupes may be used for reading and close work.

Cataracts reduce contrast and cause glare. The shorter wavelengths cause the most scatter; the color, intensity, and direction of lighting also affect glare. If a patient experiences problems in a particular lighting situation, the ophthalmologist may suggest reducing light transmission from 400–550 nm or increasing lumens directed at reading material and away from the patient's eyes.

Indications for Surgery

The most common indication for cataract surgery is the patient's desire for improved visual function. The decision is not based on a specific level of visual acuity. Rather, the patient and physician determine whether reduced visual function interferes substantially with desired activities. A detailed history is often all that is necessary to document a patient's subjective visual disability. Several questionnaires, such as the VF-14 or the Activities of Daily Vision Scale (ADVS), are available to help determine the level of impairment. Many governmental agencies and industries have minimum standards of visual function for such tasks as driving, flying, and operating complex equipment. A patient whose best-corrected visual acuity does not meet these visual requirements may need to consider cataract surgery. Once the patient has decided to seek improvement of visual function through cataract surgery, the ophthalmologist must determine, through interaction with the patient and family as well as by the results of subjective and objective testing, whether this step is advisable.

In most situations, a patient with bilateral visually significant cataracts is a candidate for surgery in the eye with the more advanced cataract. (In the very elderly, those with other contributing factors to reduced acuity, or those with severe systemic diseases, it may be appropriate to operate on the eye with better visual potential because only one eye may come to surgery.) The decision to proceed must be individualized to the patient's visual needs and potential; the same indications govern the decision to operate on the second eye. Symptomatic, surgically induced anisometropia not responsive to other nonsurgical approaches may be disabling enough to the patient to justify surgery on the second eye. A reasonable time should separate the two procedures to ensure the success and safety of the first operation before the second is undertaken.

In a patient with a monocular cataract, the decision to proceed with surgery requires carefully educating the patient regarding risks, alternatives and benefits. Common indications for surgery in this situation include loss of stereopsis, diminished peripheral vision, disabling glare, or symptomatic anisometropia. The presence of cataract in one eye directly influences driving performance and accident avoidance.

Medical indications for cataract surgery include phacolytic glaucoma, phacomorphic glaucoma, phacoantigenic uveitis, and dislocation of the lens into the anterior chamber. An additional indication is the presence of a dense cataract that obscures the view of the fundus and impedes the diagnosis or management of other ocular diseases, such as diabetic retinopathy or glaucoma.

Mangione CM, Phillips RS, Lawrence MG, et al. Improved visual function and attenuation of declines in health-related quality of life after cataract extraction. *Arch Ophthalmol.* 1994;112:1419–1425.

Owsley C, McGwin G Jr, Sloane M, et al. Impact of cataract surgery on motor vehicle crash involvement by older adults. *JAMA.* 2002;288:841–849.

Steinberg EP, Tielsch JM, Schein OD, et al. The VF–14. An index of functional impairment in patients with cataract. *Arch Ophthalmol.* 1994;112:630–638.

Preoperative Evaluation

The following evaluation and information should be obtained in order to determine if cataract surgery is warranted. The parameters suggested should be tailored to the specific patient's situation.

General Health of the Patient

A complete medical history is the starting point for the preoperative evaluation. The ophthalmic surgeon should work closely with the patient's primary care physician to achieve optimal management of all medical problems, especially diabetes mellitus, ischemic heart disease, chronic obstructive pulmonary disease, bleeding disorders, or adrenal suppression caused by systemic corticosteroids. Temporizing measures such as pharmacologic mydriasis or improved spectacle correction should be undertaken if appropriate. The ophthalmologist should be aware of any drug sensitivities and medications that might alter the outcome of surgery, such as immunosuppressants and anticoagulants. Medication allergies should be documented and patients questioned regarding sedative, narcotic, anesthetic, iodine, or latex sensitivity. Awareness of musculoskeletal disorders that limit the patient's ability to lie comfortably on the operating room table may facilitate preoperative arrangements permitting uncomplicated surgery.

Pertinent Ocular History

The ocular history will help the ophthalmologist identify conditions that could affect either the surgical approach or the visual prognosis. A history of trauma, inflammation, amblyopia, glaucoma, optic nerve abnormalities, or retinal disease can affect the visual prognosis. Past records may document the patient's visual acuity prior to the development of cataract. If the patient has had cataract surgery in the fellow eye, it is important to obtain information about the operative and postoperative course. If problems such as elevated IOP, vitreous loss, cystoid macular edema, endophthalmitis, or hemorrhage occurred in the first operation, the surgical approach and postoperative follow-up may often be modified for the second operation to reduce the risk of similar complications.

If the patient has had refractive surgery, it is helpful to obtain information about the type of procedure, original refraction, original keratometry, intraoperative complications that might have occurred, and whether the postoperative refraction is stable. This information is useful both in predicting the IOL power and in determining the surgical approach.

Social History

The decision to undertake cataract surgery is not based on the patient's visual acuity alone but rather on the effect of reduced visual function on the individual. The social history is important for documenting the patient's subjective visual disability. The surgeon should also be aware of the patient's occupation, lifestyle, and any possible chemical dependencies, including nicotine and illicit (recreational) drugs, as they relate to the postoperative recovery.

Planning Postoperative Care

In planning cataract surgery, the surgeon should evaluate the patient's ability to participate in postoperative care. The surgeon, patient, and any associated caregivers should discuss the patient's ability to administer eyedrops, maintain good ocular and general hygiene, and keep postoperative appointments. The patient also needs to understand the importance of activity restrictions in the immediate postoperative period, which may vary with the patient's lifestyle or type of surgery. (The advent of small-incision surgery has greatly minimized activity limitations.) The surgeon should assess the patient's ability to function with only the fellow eye in case visual rehabilitation is prolonged. Involvement of the patient's family or support systems preoperatively can be of considerable assistance to the patient during the postoperative period.

External Examination

The preoperative evaluation of a patient with cataract should include the body habitus and any abnormalities of the external eye and ocular adnexa. Such conditions as extensive supraclavicular fat, kyphosis, ankylosing spondylitis, generalized obesity, or head tremor may have an effect on surgical approach.

The ophthalmologist should examine the eye specifically for the presence of enophthalmos or prominent brow. Surgical approach and anesthesia may need to be altered if these conditions are present. Any entropion, ectropion, or abnormalities of eyelid closure should be treated prior to cataract surgery. Blepharitis, as manifested by collarettes, marginal eyelid thickening, and inspissation of meibomian gland secretions, should be diagnosed and treated before cataract surgery. The tear film should be examined for abnormalities in the aqueous or lipid layer, and abnormal tear dynamics, exposure keratitis, or decreased corneal sensation should be noted and treated as indicated. Nasolacrimal disease should be identified and corrected prior to surgery, particularly if there is a history of periodic inflammation, infection, or obstruction.

Motility

The clinician should evaluate ocular alignment and test the range of movement of the extraocular muscles. Cover testing should be performed to document any muscle deviation. The presence of an abnormality may suggest preexisting strabismus with amblyopia as a cause of visual loss. A significant tropia from disruption of fusion may result in diplopia following surgery; the patient must be made aware of this possibility.

Pupils

Evaluation of the pupillary response to light and accommodation is important. In addition to checking direct and consensual constriction of the pupil to light, the ophthalmologist should perform a swinging-flashlight test to detect a relative afferent pupillary defect that would indicate serious retinal or optic nerve dysfunction. Some patients with a relative afferent pupillary defect in the cataractous eye may still have improved visual function following cataract surgery; however, the patient must be informed that this test result indicates reduced visual potential.

Oval lenses and small-optic IOLs may be inappropriate for a patient who has a large pupil in moderate or dim illumination, because the edge of the optic may be exposed under these circumstances and cause glare or dysphotopsias. Further, it is helpful to assess the pupillary size after dilation: pupils that are fibrotic or have pseudoexfoliation syndrome may not dilate well and may increase the surgical risk. Foreknowledge of these conditions allows the surgeon to prepare appropriately and alter the surgical technique as necessary for a safer procedure.

Slit-Lamp Examination

Conjunctiva

The conjunctiva is examined for the presence of scarring, filtering blebs, or lack of mobility over the sclera. Symblepharon or shortening of the fornices could be associated with underlying systemic or ocular surface diseases. These special conditions may limit surgical exposure or indicate a clear corneal approach. Vascularization or scarring from previous chemical injury or previous ocular surgery, including refractive surgery, may dictate changes in the surgical approach.

Cornea

To evaluate the cornea before cataract surgery, the clinician should assess corneal thickness and look for the presence of guttata. When possible, specular reflection with the slit lamp may provide an estimate of the endothelial cell count and morphology. Marked abnormalities of the endothelial layer or a thickness greater than 640 µm, as measured by pachymetry, secondary to stromal edema suggests a poor prognosis for corneal clarity following cataract surgery. Although such conditions are not contraindications to surgery, it is important to discuss them, as well as the possibility of combined or subsequent corneal surgery, with the patient. The ophthalmologist should tailor the surgery to minimize trauma to the endothelium. Irregularity of Descemet's membrane associated with corneal guttata, as seen at the slit lamp, may limit visual potential. In addition, long-term contact lens wearers and patients with a previous history of dystrophy, superficial punctate keratitis, arcus, or chlamydial infection may have pannus or stromal opacities that may limit the surgical view during cataract extraction.

The proliferation of refractive surgery procedures has implications for planning cataract surgery. For example, it is helpful to obtain the original keratometry readings prior to refractive surgery, if possible. In addition, corneal topography is useful in evaluating the contour of the cornea for irregular astigmatism and for more precise keratometry readings. Special techniques for IOL power calculation and selection may need to be made (see Chapter 10 for further discussion). It is important to identify any weakened or thinned areas in the cornea that may need to be avoided during surgery.

Anterior Chamber

A shallow anterior chamber may indicate anatomically narrow angles, nanophthalmos, an intumescent lens, or forward displacement by posterior pathology (for example, a ciliary body tumor). Knowing the anterior chamber depth and measurement of the axial thickness of the lens nucleus may help the surgeon plan the wound size for extracapsular cataract extraction (ECCE) or choose between ECCE and phacoemulsification.

Preoperative gonioscopy should rule out angle abnormalities, including the presence of peripheral anterior synechiae, neovascularization, or a prominent major arterial circle. Use of a 3-mirror lens may help in evaluating the lens zonule for traumatic or genetic dehiscence. Gonioscopy is essential if anterior chamber IOL implantation is anticipated. The ophthalmologist should note the presence of peripheral anterior synechiae or abnormal iris vessels to determine if angle implant fixation is possible.

Iris

As discussed in the preceding sections, the clinician should check the pupil size and note the presence of synechiae after dilation. Radial iridotomy, sector iridectomy, posterior synechiolysis, sphincterotomy, or iris retraction may be necessary to provide adequate exposure during surgery if the pupil dilates poorly.

Crystalline Lens

The appearance of the lens should be carefully noted, both before and after dilation of the pupil. The visual significance of oil droplet nuclear cataracts and small PSCs is best appreciated before dilation of the pupil. After dilation, nuclear density can be evaluated, exfoliation syndrome can be detected, and opacities and distortion of the retinoscopic reflex will be easier to visualize.

The clarity of the media in the visual axis should be evaluated to assess the lenticular contribution to the visual deficit. A thin slit beam of white light is focused on the posterior capsule. The light is then changed to cobalt blue; if the posterior capsule is no longer illuminated (as a result of blue-light scatter), the contribution of the lens opacity to visual acuity is most often 20/50 or worse. Relatively small PSCs may cause surprisingly severe visual loss; conversely, even dense brunescent nuclear sclerotic cataracts may allow remarkably good visual acuity, especially at near.

The position of the lens and integrity of the zonular fibers must also be evaluated. Decentration of the lens, phacodonesis, or excessive distance between the lens and pupillary margin may indicate subluxation of the lens as a result of previous trauma, metabolic disorders, or hypermature cataract. An indentation or flattening of the lens periphery may indicate focal loss of zonular support.

Limitations of Slit-Lamp Examination

Some visually significant cataracts may appear nearly normal upon slit-lamp biomicroscopy. Examination of the lens with the retinoscope, however, may reveal cataract-induced visual changes. By examining the retinoscopic reflex, the clinician may detect posterior subcapsular opacities, refractile nuclear changes, or even diffuse cataracts. Similarly, examination using the direct ophthalmoscope through the +10 D lens at a distance of 2 feet will enhance the portions of the cataractous lens that are producing optical aberrations. This technique is particularly useful in identifying oil droplet cataracts.

Fundus Evaluation

Ophthalmoscopy

Both direct and indirect ophthalmoscopy should be undertaken to evaluate the anatomical integrity of the posterior segment. The indirect ophthalmoscope is not useful for judging the visual significance of cataract. Although the direct ophthalmoscope is more useful in judging media clarity, the examiner must keep in mind that it, too, provides light that is more intense than that available to the patient under ambient lighting conditions. A full fundus examination is necessary to evaluate the macula, optic nerve, retinal vessels, and retinal periphery. Particular attention should be paid to early macular degeneration, which may limit visual rehabilitation after an otherwise uneventful cataract extraction.

Patients with diabetes should be examined carefully for the presence of macular edema or retinal ischemia, with or without neovascularization. Retinal ischemia may progress to posterior or anterior neovascularization, especially if the surgeon uses an intracapsular technique or ruptures the posterior capsule during extracapsular surgery. Careful examination of the retinal periphery may reveal the presence of vitreoretinal traction, lattice degeneration, or preexisting retinal holes that may warrant preoperative treatment. Intracapsular surgery and primary discission of the posterior capsule are associated with a significantly higher incidence of retinal detachment and cystoid macular edema.

Optic Nerve

The optic nerve should be examined for pallor, cup–disc ratio, and any abnormalities. Visual acuity, confrontation visual field testing, measurement of intraocular pressure, and pupillary examination will also indicate if more formal testing may be needed.

Fundus Evaluation With Opaque Media

If the cataract prevents direct visualization of the posterior segment of the eye, other methods may be used to evaluate the retina. B-scan ultrasonography of the posterior pole of the eye is useful whenever it is impossible to view the retina. This technique can help determine the preoperative status of the posterior segment by elucidating whether retinal detachment, vitreous opacities, posterior pole tumor, or staphyloma is present. (See also BCSC Section 3, *Clinical Optics.*) Light projection, 2-point discrimination, gross color vision, Maddox rod projection, or the presence of entoptic phenomena may also be useful in detecting retinal pathology. Electroretinography (ERG) and visual evoked response (VER) are also helpful in specific circumstances (see Special Tests later in this chapter).

Measurements of Visual Function

Visual Acuity Testing

Visual acuity testing in the ophthalmologist's office is commonly performed in a darkened room. Because decreased Snellen acuity from a visually significant cataract may occasionally be demonstrated only in a lighted room, it can be helpful to check visual acuity in both light and dark conditions. It is also important to test distance and near visual acuity and to perform a careful refraction to determine best-corrected visual acuity. With some patients, pinhole visual acuity is better than that obtained with best refractive correction. Visual acuity may improve after pupillary dilation, especially in patients with PSC.

Brightness Acuity

When a patient complains of glare, it is important to test distance and near visual acuity in a well-lighted room. Testing can be done with a nonprojected eye chart in ambient light conditions or with a projected eye chart and an off-axis bright light directed at the patient. A variety of instruments is available to standardize and facilitate this measurement. Patients with significant cataracts commonly show a decrease of 3 or more lines under these conditions, compared with the results when visual acuity is tested in the dark.

Contrast Sensitivity

Various methods and instruments have been developed to test contrast sensitivity in the ophthalmologist's office. A wide variety of instruments and charts is available to test contrast sensitivity in the clinical setting. Patients with cataracts may experience diminished contrast sensitivity even when Snellen acuity is preserved. (See also BCSC Section 3, *Clinical Optics.*)

Visual Field Testing

Confrontation visual fields should be tested. Patients with a history of glaucoma, optic nerve disease, or retinal abnormality may benefit from Goldmann or automated visual field testing to document the degree of preoperative visual field loss. In patients with optically dense cataracts that block the view of the retinal periphery, light projection may be helpful to test the peripheral visual field. Visual field testing may help the ophthalmologist to identify visual loss resulting from other disease processes. However, preoperative visual field loss does not preclude improvement in visual function following cataract surgery, and lens opacities may make formal visual fields less reliable.

Special Tests

Potential Acuity Estimation

Potential acuity estimation can be helpful in assessing the lenticular contribution to visual loss. Laser interferometry and the potential acuity meter are two of several methods by which potential acuity can be estimated.

In *laser interferometry,* twin sources of monochromatic helium–neon laser light create a diffraction fringe pattern on the retinal surface. Transmission of this pattern is mostly independent of lens opacities. It is possible to estimate retinal visual acuity by varying the spacing of the fringe; however, the area of the pattern subtending the retina is considerably larger than the fovea. For this reason, small foveal lesions that limit visual acuity may not be detected.

The *potential acuity meter* projects a numerical or Snellen vision chart through a small entrance pupil. The image can be projected into the eye around lenticular opacities.

Laser interferometry and potential acuity meter determinations can be useful in estimating visual acuity before cataract extraction. Both are much more predictive in eyes with moderate lens opacities than in those with severe lens opacities. In addition, these tests can be misleading in the presence of several disorders, including age-related macular degeneration, amblyopia, macular edema, glaucoma, small macular scars, and serous retinal detachment. An accurate clinical examination of the eye is as good a predictor of the visual outcome as laser interferometry or potential acuity testing.

Fish GE, Birch DG, Fuller DG, et al. A comparison of visual function tests in eyes with maculopathy. *Ophthalmology.* 1986;93:1177–1182.

Miller ST, Graney MJ, Elam JT, et al. Predictions of outcomes from cataract surgery in elderly persons. *Ophthalmology.* 1988;95:1125–1129.

Tests of Macular Function

Because cataracts can obstruct the view of the fundus, direct examination may be difficult. The following tests measure function rather than appearance.

Maddox rod

In patients with dense cataracts that preclude adequate visualization of the fundus pre-operatively, Maddox rod testing can be used to grossly evaluate macular function. Any large scotoma, represented as a loss of the red line as viewed by the patient, should raise the possibility of significant macular disease. (See also BCSC Section 3, *Clinical Optics*, on cylindrical lenses.)

Photostress recovery test

The photostress recovery time can be used to estimate macular function. After a penlight is shined directly into a normal eye (the "photostress"), a recovery period is necessary before the patient can identify the Snellen letters 1 line larger than that individual's baseline visual acuity (the photostress recovery time). Normal photostress recovery time averages 27 seconds with a standard deviation of 11 seconds. Photostress recovery time is 50 seconds or less in 99% of normal eyes. Prolonged photostress recovery time is an indication of macular disease.

Glaser JS, Savino PJ, Sumers KD, et al. The photostress recovery test in the clinical assessment of visual function. *Am J Ophthalmol*. 1977;83:255–260.

Blue-light entoptoscopy

During a blue-light entoptoscopy examination, the patient is asked to view an intense, homogeneous blue-light background. Under these conditions, the white blood cells coursing through the perifoveal capillaries produce shadows. If the patient sees the shadows, macular function is probably intact. However, this test has limited utility because many patients find the instructions difficult to comprehend.

Loebl M, Riva CE. Macular circulation and the flying corpuscles phenomenon. *Ophthalmology*. 1978;85:911–917.

Sinclair SH, Loebl M, Riva CE. Blue field entoptic phenomenon in cataract patients. *Arch Ophthalmol*. 1979;97:1092–1095.

Purkinje's entoptic phenomenon

Purkinje's entoptic phenomenon test is also subjective. A rapidly oscillating point source of light is shined through the patient's closed eyelids. The patient's ability to detect shadow images of his or her retinal vasculature provides a very rough indication that the retina is attached.

Electroretinography (ERG) and visual evoked response (VER)

In rare cases where other testing is inconclusive, ERG or VER testing can be done to evaluate retinal and/or optic nerve function. These tests are discussed fully in BCSC Section 12, *Retina and Vitreous*.

Preoperative Measurements

Several measurements, discussed in the following sections, should be taken preoperatively, especially if the surgeon plans to implant an IOL.

Refraction

Careful refraction must be performed on both eyes. This assessment is useful in planning the IOL power necessary to obtain the postoperative refraction desired by the patient and the ophthalmologist. If the fellow eye has a clear lens and a high refractive error that requires spectacle correction, obtaining a similar refractive result in the operated eye may avoid problems with postoperative anisometropia. These problems may also be avoided if a contact lens can be successfully worn in the phakic eye. If the fellow eye has a cataract or if the patient expresses a desire to see at a distance or at near without spectacle correction, however, it may be preferable to plan the implant power to achieve postoperative emmetropia.

Biometry

In order to calculate the appropriate IOL power, the eye's axial length must be accurately measured through A-scan ultrasonography or optical coherence biometry. In addition, corneal power must be determined through keratometry or corneal topography. (IOL power determination is discussed in greater detail in Chapter 8.)

Corneal topography

Corneal topography is a method for mapping the corneal contour. It uses a method similar to the Placido disk or it uses elevation mapping and gives more information about corneal power than manual keratometry does. Irregular astigmatism and subclinical keratoconus are more readily diagnosed by topography. Corneal topography is particularly helpful if the patient has previously undergone keratorefractive surgery, if a toric IOL may be implanted, or if the surgeon plans to perform astigmatic keratotomy at the same time as cataract extraction.

Corneal Pachymetry

Corneal pachymetry, a measurement of corneal thickness, is useful in assessing the function of the endothelium. Pachymeters are available in two types: optical and ultrasonic. Ultrasonic pachymeters are generally more reliable than optical pachymeters and can be used to estimate corneal endothelial cell function by measuring corneal thickness. In general, central corneal thickness greater than 640 μm in patients with endothelial dysfunction is consistent with corneal edema and increases the likelihood of postoperative decreased corneal clarity.

Specular Microscopy

Specular microscopy of corneal endothelial cells is used to determine the number of cells per square millimeter. Normal endothelial cell counts are greater than 2400 cells/mm^2. Because cataract surgery causes some loss of endothelial cells, the risk of postoperative corneal decompensation following surgery is increased if preoperative endothelial cell counts are low.

Endothelial cell morphology, including enlargement (polymegethism) and irregularity (pleomorphism), provides additional information about the cornea's ability to withstand stress. (See BCSC Section 8, *External Disease and Cornea*.)

Patient Preparation and Informed Consent

The patient should have a clear understanding of the risks and benefits of cataract surgery. The surgeon and patient should discuss

- the indications for and alternatives to surgery, as well as the likelihood of significant visual improvement
- the risk of common operative and postoperative complications
- the anticipated time course for activity limitations and reasonable expectations for the patient's return to regular daily activities
- the role of preexisting ocular and medical disorders on visual outcome
- the desired postoperative refractive status and the limitations of pseudophakic correction
- when the final optical correction will be given
- the frequency and duration of postoperative eye medications

If patients and their caregivers are adequately prepared prior to surgery, they can anticipate a routine postoperative course and understand problems that may develop. It is helpful to include a family member or friend in these preoperative discussions so the patient is able to refresh his or her memory. Written or audiovisual materials may also help.

> *Cataract in the Adult Eye*. Preferred Practice Pattern. San Francisco: American Academy of Ophthalmology; 2001.

CHAPTER 8

Surgery for Cataract

Historical Development of Cataract Surgery

Ancient surgeons did not recognize that the cataract was in fact the opacified crystalline lens. Rather, they considered it a "suffusion" that formed between the pupil and the lens. Early writings of Celsus (25 BC–AD 50) alluded to the fact that some practitioners (Philoxenes, 300 BC) surgically treated cataract, but any records and descriptions of their work have been lost. The term *cataract* was introduced by Constantinus Africanus (AD 1010–1087), a Carthaginian monk and ocularist, who translated the Arabic term for suffusion into the Latin *cataracta*, meaning a "waterfall" or "blockage of flow," such as the cataracts that impeded navigation of the Nile River.

Couching

The surgical treatment of cataract is an ancient art that spans 2 millennia. Surgeons in ancient India practiced couching as early as 800 BC (Fig 8-1). Couching was performed by a surgeon who sat facing the patient, whose face would be illuminated by bright sun streaming in through a window. An assistant was positioned behind the patient to stabilize the patient's head. A pointed needle was plunged either through the sclera 4 mm temporal to the limbus or through clear cornea. Pharmacologic dilation was not possible. The surgeon had to be ambidextrous enough to hold the lancet in the right hand for the left eye and vice versa. The needle was passed through the conjunctiva and sclera in a blind approach behind the iris toward the lens. Little did ancient surgeons realize that they had established the modern pars plana approach. The surgeon would then use a blunted needle to push the white opacity downward or backward. During these maneuvers, the patient would move the eye medially or superiorly to further wiggle the lens from its zonular fibers. The proof of success was the ability of the patient to see forms and figures again.

Ammar, an Iraqi ocularist (AD 996–1020), described the suction of a soft cataract through a hollow needle. Syrians in the 12th and 13th centuries also tried this aspiration method, which flourished for a while but then fell into disregard.

In the Middle Ages, it was considered undignified and barbarous to practice surgery, and couchers were held in disrepute. Itinerant couchers traveled from town to town to offer their services, and they would use a common sewing needle to couch cataracts in the village square (Fig 8-2). The complication rates were high, and a couching procedure was considered a success if the patient was able to ambulate without assistance.

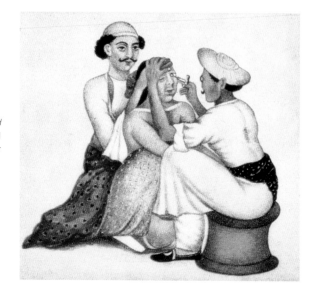

Figure 8-1 Couching. *(Reproduced from Duke-Elder S.* Diseases of the Lens and Vitreous; Glaucoma and Hypotony. *St Louis: Mosby; 1969.)*

Early Extracapsular Extraction Procedures

An advancement in the development of cataract surgery was *extracting* the cataract from the eye, rather than just displacing it by couching. Jacques Daviel (1696–1762), a Frenchman, published the first account of cataract extraction through the pupil and out of the eye through a limbal incision. An incision was made through the inferior cornea and enlarged with scissors. The cornea was elevated, the lens capsule incised, the nucleus expressed, and cortex removed by curettage (Fig 8-3). Each operation took 4 minutes and was performed without either anesthesia or aseptic technique.

Daviel's extracapsular cataract extraction (ECCE) was an innovation and an improvement over couching, but the technique had some significant drawbacks that limited its wide acceptance. Endophthalmitis was not infrequent. Because the cortex removal was incomplete, chronic inflammation, secondary capsular opacification, and pupillary-block glaucoma were potential complications. Uveal prolapse sometimes occurred because the wound was unstable. In addition, because the procedure was performed most safely after the cortex had liquefied, the patient had to wait until the cataract was "ripe."

A German ophthalmologist, Albrecht von Graefe (1828–1870), improved upon extracapsular technique with the development of a knife that created a better-apposed wound. This innovation decreased the rate of infection and uveal prolapse, and extracapsular extraction gained more acceptance.

Early Intracapsular Extraction Procedures

Because of the drawbacks of extracapsular extraction, techniques were sought that would remove the cataractous lens in its entirety from the eye. Samuel Sharp, who expressed a cataractous lens, capsule intact, through a limbal incision using pressure from his thumb, was among the first to successfully perform intracapsular cataract extraction (ICCE). He practiced this method in London in 1753.

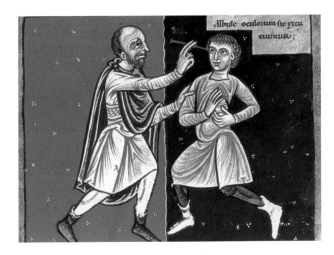

Figure 8-2 Couching. *(Reproduced from Wertenbaker L. The Eye: Window to the World. New York: Torstar Books; 1984.)*

One of the chief problems to be solved in the development of ICCE was how to lyse or break the zonular fibers. Colonel Henry Smith, an Englishman stationed in India, used external manipulation with a muscle hook to mechanically break the inferior attachments. He then used the muscle hook to expel the cataractous lens from the eye through a limbal wound. The lens would "tumble"; that is, the inferior pole of the lens would exit the eye before the superior pole. His technique, called the *Smith-Indian operation,* was used in 50,000 cases over a 25-year period at the end of the 19th century and beginning of the 20th century.

Another method of zonular disintegration and lens removal was traction. Toothless forceps, developed by ophthalmologists such as Frederick Verhoeff and Jean Baptiste Kalt, were used to grasp the lens capsule (Fig 8-4). The cataract was then gently pulled from the eye using a side-to-side motion that broke the zonular insertion. Suction cup–like devices called *erysiphakes* were devised by Stoewer and by Ignacio Barraquer (1884–1965) to remove the lens with traction (Fig 8-5).

Tadeusz Krwawicz in Poland first developed a cryoprobe in 1961. This instrument would form an iceball, fusing the lens capsule, cortex, and nucleus, and lessening the risk of capsule rupture as the cataract was removed from the eye. (Figure 8-11 shows a modern cryoprobe.) Chemical dissolution of the zonular fibers with the enzyme alpha-chymotrypsin was first reported by Joaquin Barraquer in 1957. Its use enhanced the safety of ICCE by increasing the ease of lens removal.

ICCE evolved into a very successful operation. By 1944, 85% of patients in published series had a postoperative best-corrected visual acuity of 20/30 or better, a substantial improvement over couching and early extracapsular technique. However, there remained a 5% rate of potentially blinding complications, including infection, hemorrhage, retinal detachment, and cystoid macular edema. In addition, the problems of optically rehabilitating the aphakic patient with glasses remained formidable.

Blodi FC. Cataract surgery. In: Albert DM, Edwards DD, eds. *The History of Ophthalmology.* Cambridge, MA: Blackwell Scientific; 1996:165–177.

Gorin G. *History of Ophthalmology.* New York: Raven Press; 1982.

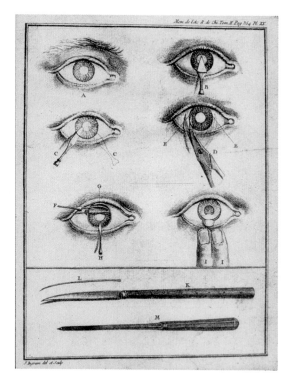

Figure 8-3 Daviel J. Sur une nouvelle methode de guérir la cataracte par l'extraction du cristalin. *(From Louis M, et al. Memoires de l'Académie Royale de Chirurgie. Paris: Théophile Barrois Lejeune; 1787.)*

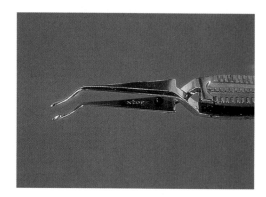

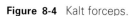

Figure 8-4 Kalt forceps.

Modern Extracapsular Techniques

A shift from ICCE procedures to new methods of ECCE technique evolved in an effort to decrease the rate of potentially blinding complications and to facilitate the placement of intraocular lenses. By leaving the posterior lens capsule intact, the surgeon could reduce the risk of vitreous loss and the potentially blinding complications of retinal detachment, cystoid macular edema, and aphakic bullous keratopathy. Key to the development and acceptance of modern ECCE technique was the growing use of operating microscopes for increased magnification and improved methods of cortical removal, as well as the ability to deal with posterior capsular opacification.

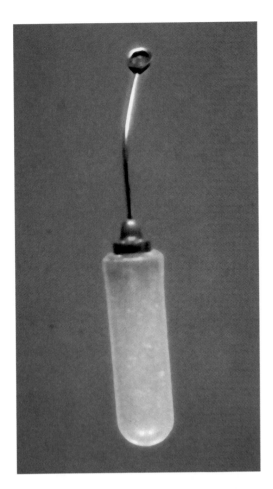

Figure 8-5 Barraquer erysiphake.

Initially, all extracapsular techniques involved nuclear expression, but in 1967 Charles Kelman of New York developed phacoemulsification. This new type of ECCE ultrasonically emulsified the lens nucleus, allowing the operation to be performed through a smaller incision. Phacoemulsification has continued to grow in popularity as techniques and instrumentation have become more refined; it is now the dominant method for cataract removal in the United States.

Anesthesia for Cataract Surgery

Historical Considerations

Historically, cataract surgery was performed without anesthesia. Karl Koller used topical cocaine anesthesia of the limbus in the late 1800s. Retrobulbar anesthesia was first described in 1884 by Herman Knapp, who injected 4% cocaine for ocular anesthesia prior to enucleation surgery. The modern technique of retrobulbar anesthesia, described in 1945 by Walter Atkinson, remains a commonly used technique for intraocular surgery.

Other issues that may arise during preoperative preparation include routine systemic antibiotic prophylaxis and anticoagulation therapy. *Systemic antibiotics* for the prevention of bacterial endocarditis or bacteremia in those patients with artifical heart valves or mitral valve prolapse are not recommended in the event of elective intraocular surgery. Cataract surgery is not considered to be an invasive procedure that induces transient bacteremia, and therefore antibiotic prophylaxis is not required. This fact may be generalized to joint prostheses as well. *Anticoagulation therapy* should be maintained in those individuals at high risk for a thromboembolic event if their oral anticoagulant is discontinued. Topical anesthesia is a major advantage in promoting a safer operation for these patients.

Dajani AS, Taubert KA, Wilson W, et al. Prevention of bacterial endocarditis: recommendations by the American Heart Association. *JAMA.* 1997;277:1794–1801.

Kearon C, Hirsh J. Management of anticoagulation before and after elective surgery. *N Engl J Med.* 1997;336:1506–1511.

Liesegang TJ. Perioperative antibiotic prophylaxis in cataract surgery. *Cornea.* 1999;18:383–402.

Liesegang TJ. Prophylactic antibiotics in cataract operations. *Mayo Clin Proc.* 1997;72:149–159.

Menikoff JA, Speaker MG, Marmor M, et al. A case-control study of risk factors for postoperative endophthalmitis. *Ophthalmology.* 1991;98:1761–1768.

Speaker MG, Menikoff JA. Prophylaxis of endophthalmitis with topical povidone-iodine. *Ophthalmology.* 1991;98:1769–1775.

Srinivasan R, Tiroumal S, Kanungo R, et al. Microbial contamination of the anterior chamber during phacoemulsification. *J Cataract and Refract Surg.* 2002;28:2173–2176.

Theory of Wound Construction for Cataract Surgery

Historically, cataract wounds were created with a long, tapered blade (von Graefe knife) inserted from the temporal limbus across the anterior chamber and out the nasal limbus (ab externo). The blade would then cut superiorly, exiting with a flap of conjunctiva still attached to the superior corneal edge. After the lens was extracted by capsule forceps, the patient's head was maintained in a fixed position with sandbags for a week or more to allow this 180° wound to self-seal. If the wound had been made perfectly and the edges reapposed without incarcerating iris or vitreous, it was possible for this type of wound to seal itself without sutures. Later in the evolution of this procedure, silk sutures were placed across the wound, progressing in number from 1 to 9 or more as the quality of the silk and needles improved. The sandbags were retired.

Unfortunately, the frequency of wound complications was quite high with these early techniques. Flat anterior chambers were common during the first postoperative week, and secondary aphakic glaucoma with broad peripheral anterior synechiae often followed. Filtering blebs, high against-the-rule astigmatism, and wound leaks with endophthalmitis resulted when wound closure was defective. The development of the surgical microscope and fine needles and suture materials enabled the surgeon to observe the wound edges and secure them precisely. These improvements reduced morbidity drastically and made possible the early ambulation of patients following cataract extraction.

Single-Plane Incisions

The traditional intracapsular cataract incision and, to some extent, the extracapsular cataract incision produce straight-entry incisions that directly enter the anterior chamber. Watertight closure of these incisions necessitates deep radial suture bites to reapproximate the wound edges. These radial sutures compress tissue and cause flattening over the wound, which results in steepening of the central cornea and with-the-rule astigmatism.

Following a straight-entry incision for either ICCE or ECCE, the patient typically waited 6–8 weeks to allow the suture-induced wound distortion to fade before receiving aphakic spectacles. Sutures were often cut or removed prior to dispensing the final prescription for glasses in order to reduce the keratometric and refractive cylinder. The widespread use of IOLs, however, has given patients the expectation of good vision almost immediately following surgery. With the advent of phacoemulsification and small-incision IOLs, the wound has become smaller. These developments make more rapid visual recovery possible by minimizing or eliminating suture-induced astigmatism.

Scleral Tunnel Incisions

Small, posteriorly placed cataract incisions reduce the incidence of induced with-the-rule astigmatism in the initial postoperative period as well as long-term against-the-rule astigmatism. Lower induced astigmatism in the immediate postoperative period is associated with faster recovery of visual acuity, and lower induced astigmatism over time is associated with a more stable refraction and better uncorrected vision. Therefore, smaller and more posteriorly placed incisions have some advantages over larger, more anteriorly positioned cataract incisions. The superiorly placed scleral tunnel incision with an internal corneal lip is a frequently used incision among cataract surgeons.

Moving the entry incision more posteriorly and creating a longer tunnel with a beveled entry wound into the anterior chamber enhances the valve effect of the wound closure and increases the likelihood of achieving a self-sealing wound. The architecture of the wound and the delicate handling of tissue edges are critical for creating the valve effect that successfully closes the wound. This valve effect is not reliable if the eye is soft: adequate intraocular pressure is needed to maintain wound apposition, so the surgeon must restore the IOP at the end of surgery.

The closure of a step or tunnel incision depends not on radial compression of the anterior and posterior lips of the wound but rather on reapproximation of the surfaces of the tunnel flap. Scleral incision closure technique has included radial sutures (Figs 8-9 and 8-10A) as well as horizontal sutures (Figs 8-10B,C), which can seal the cataract wound without causing high degrees of with-the-rule astigmatism and its associated delays in visual recovery.

With the continuing evolution of techniques for self-sealing wounds, many surgeons have elected not to suture the wound at all. Long-term evaluation of the results and stability of this type of wound closure seem to indicate that small scleral tunnel and clear corneal incisions, both with and without suture closure, are relatively stable and induce minimal astigmatism. Even though no-stitch cataract surgery has many advantages, the surgeon should always be ready to place a suture if any aspect of the wound closure appears to be inadequate.

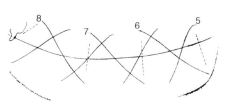

Figure 8-9 The shoelace suture. *(Reproduced by permission from Maloney WF, Grindle L. Textbook of Phacoemulsification. Fallbrook, CA: Lasenda; 1988.)*

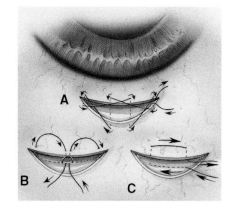

Figure 8-10 Wound closure techniques. **A**, Classic radial running x-closure must be keratometrically monitored (preferably quantitatively rather than qualitatively) during tying to avoid undesired postoperative astigmatism. Alternatively, horizontal suturing techniques using multiple bites **(B)** or a single bite **(C)** have been devised to try to decrease the induced astigmatism. *(Reproduced with permission from Johnson SH. Phacoemulsification. Focal Points: Clinical Modules for Ophthalmologists. San Francisco: American Academy of Ophthalmology; 1994, module 6. Illustration by Christine Gralapp.)*

Potential complications of inadequate wound closure include those from the early days of cataract surgery: filtering blebs, late-onset against-the-rule astigmatism, and wound leaks with endophthalmitis. It is also possible for high concentrations of antibiotics, injected subconjunctivally at the end of surgery, to reflux into the anterior chamber with toxic results.

The techniques and procedures for making a scleral tunnel incision are discussed later in this chapter under Types of Cataract Surgery: Extracapsular Extraction by Phacoemulsification in the subsection Procedure, Incisions.

Clear Corneal Incisions

Clear corneal incisions are gaining in popularity, especially for phacoemulsification with topical anesthesia. These small incisions are typically 2.7–4.0 mm wide, just large enough to accommodate the foldable IOL. They usually have little or no effect on preexisting astigmatism. One technique for clear corneal surgery involves a grooved or biplanar incision that is theoretically more watertight, whereas others use a single-plane entry. Some surgeons believe that a grooved or biplanar corneal incision is more likely to affect astigmatism. The deeper the vertical groove, the more likely it is to function as a peripheral astigmatic keratotomy (AK) incision by flattening the cornea in that meridian. Some surgeons place the clear corneal incisions in the meridian of the plus cylinder in hopes of reducing the astigmatism. Other surgeons find these incisions to be astigmatically neutral and prefer temporal incisions in all cases. The latter surgeons may use limbal relaxing incisions (LRIs) to reduce preexisting astigmatism (see Theory of Wound Construction for Cataract Surgery, Modification of Preexisting Astigmatism).

The clear corneal incision technique has a number of advantages:

- It is well suited for topical anesthesia, which brings its own set of advantages.
- It avoids vascular tissue with the risk of bleeding [particularly beneficial in patients on chronic anticoagulation (eg, warfarin) or antiplatelet (eg, aspirin) therapy].
- It reduces the risk of postoperative hyphema.
- It creates a self-sealing wound that does not usually require sutures and allows for rapid visual rehabilitation.
- It offers better accessibility because brow obstruction is eliminated with a temporal approach.
- It offers better red reflex.
- It eliminates the conjunctival incision, which shortens the procedure and preserves the conjunctiva for future surgery (eg, filtering procedures).
- It has minimal or no effect on astigmatism.

However, the surgeon should also be aware of the disadvantages of clear corneal cataract surgery, which include the following:

- greater degree of technical difficulty
- need for the surgeon to adapt to a different surgical position
- lack of forehead support for the surgeon's hands
- need to enlarge the incision for use of nonfoldable IOLs
- difficulty in converting to a manual expression ECCE technique
- potential for greater endothelial cell loss as a result of the proximity of the phaco tip to the peripheral cornea
- possible corneal thermal burns
- higher incidence of endophthalmitis in some studies

Specific surgical techniques for clear corneal incisions are discussed later in this chapter under Types of Cataract Surgery: Extracapsular Extraction by Phacoemulsification in the subsection Procedure, Incisions.

Eisner G, Schneider P, Telger TC. *Eye Surgery: An Introduction to Operative Technique.* 2nd ed. New York: Springer-Verlag; 1990.

Masket S. Cataract incision and closure. *Focal Points: Clinical Modules for Ophthalmologists.* San Francisco: American Academy of Ophthalmology; 1995, module 3.

Masket S. Horizontal anchor suture closure method for small incision cataract surgery. *J Cataract Refract Surg.* 1991;17(suppl):689–695.

Nagaki Y, Hayasaka S, Kadoi C, et al Bacterial endophthalmitis after small-incision cataract surgery: effect of incision placement and intraocular lens type. *J Cataract Refract Surg.* 2003;29:20–26.

of the lens without iris trauma. The use of orbital massage and/or osmotic agents (for example, mannitol, glycerin, isosorbide) prior to surgery can minimize vitreous prolapse during cataract extraction and facilitate implantation of an angle-supported IOL. Following administration of the local anesthetic, orbital massage is performed by intermittent digital pressure on the closed eyelids or by use of an oculopressive device such as a Honan balloon, mercury bag, or sponge ball and strap. Massage helps to distribute the anesthetic agent within the orbit, reduce orbital volume and pressure on the globe, and lower the IOP. Osmotic agents are used less frequently because of problems associated with volume load in patients with heart or kidney failure and occasional nausea or urinary urgency during surgery under local anesthesia.

Procedure

After inserting an eyelid speculum to part the eyelids and placing a superior bridle suture beneath the superior rectus tendon to stabilize the globe, the surgeon creates either a fornix-based or limbal-based conjunctival flap. Wet-field cautery is typically used for hemostasis. A scleral support ring may be needed in young patients or in those with high myopia to avoid scleral collapse when the lens is extracted and in patients with deep-set eyes to improve exposure.

The peripheral corneal section or limbal incision with a conjunctival flap must be large enough to accommodate the intact lens and the extraction instrument. It usually measures 160°–180° (12–14 mm length). Wound placement varies according to surgeon preference and patient need. More anterior or corneal incisions may be of shorter chord length and involve less bleeding. However, their closure induces central corneal steepening in the meridian centering the wound. More posterior incisions heal faster and, when covered by a conjunctival flap, are more comfortable to the patient. Posterior incisions induce less astigmatism and are less damaging to the corneal endothelium, but they cause more bleeding.

In general, a partial-thickness limbal groove is fashioned perpendicular to the scleral surface for 160°–180°. To facilitate rapid and precise wound closure, preplaced sutures are passed across the wound and then pulled out of the groove. If an IOL is to be inserted, the preplaced sutures are positioned across the wound, leaving a 6–7-mm gap superiorly, through which the IOL can be passed. In order to create a more secure 2-plane incision, the surgeon uses a sharp microknife to enter the anterior chamber in a beveled plane. The wound is then enlarged with either the microknife or corneoscleral scissors, while the beveled plane is maintained.

A peripheral iridectomy is routinely created for ICCE to avoid postoperative pupillary block from the intact vitreous face or from an angle-supported lens implant. An assistant may be used to elevate the corneal edge of the wound, and the iris is retracted, exposing the superior pole of the lens. A cellulose sponge is used to dry the anterior lens surface to facilitate cryoadhesion. The surgeon then places the cryoprobe on the midperiphery of the superior pole of the lens until cryoadhesion occurs. The cataract is removed through the wound by gently elevating the lens and moving it from side to side to strip the zonular attachments (Fig 8-11). If the cryoprobe becomes attached to other intraocular structures such as iris or cornea, an assistant must wet the cryoprobe with balanced

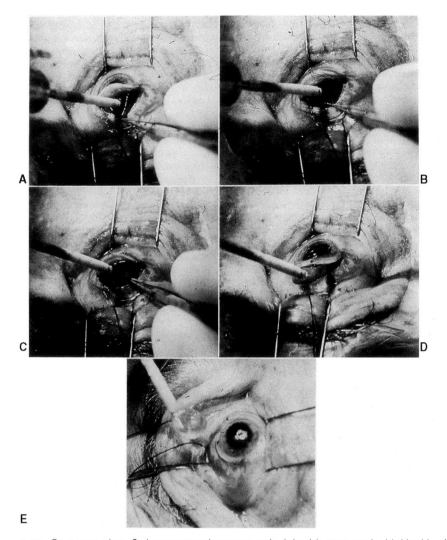

Figure 8-11 Cryoextraction. **A**, Lens rotated to surgeon's right. Iris retracted with Hoskins No. 19 forceps. **B**, Lens rotated to surgeon's left. **C**, Lens lifted. **D**, Lens slid out of eye. **E**, Extraction completed. *(Reproduced with permission from Jaffe NS, Jaffe MS, Jaffe GF. Cataract Surgery and Its Complications. 5th ed. St Louis: Mosby; 1990.)*

salt solution to break the unwanted adhesion. As the lens is extracted, the iris is reposited, and the anterior wound margin is released. The wound is then closed by pulling up and tying the preplaced sutures.

If an anterior chamber IOL is to be inserted, the pupil is constricted with either acetylcholine or carbachol, and the anterior chamber is filled with either air or viscoelastic. The injection of air is helpful to identify vitreous in the anterior chamber and may indicate the need for additional vitrectomy. The placement of a lens glide facilitates the proper placement of the anterior chamber IOL. The inferior haptic of the anterior chamber IOL is passed between the preplaced sutures into the inferior chamber angle.

A forceps or lens hook is used to place the superior IOL haptic in the superior chamber angle. The viscoelastic or air is then removed and replaced with sterile balanced salt solution, and the wound is closed with additional 10–0 nylon sutures. (See Primary Intraocular Lens Implantation in Adults later in this chapter for a more detailed discussion of IOL implantation.)

Postoperative Course

On the first postoperative day, visual acuity should be consistent with the refractive state of the eye, the clarity of the cornea and media, and the visual potential of the retina and optic nerve. If the eye has been left aphakic, it can be corrected approximately with a +10 to +12 D lens, or a +4 D lens can be used as a telescope. The surgeon should evaluate the cornea, the security of the incision, the anterior chamber depth, the degree of inflammatory reaction, and the IOP. The posterior segment should be visualized to judge vitreous clarity and position and to note any retinal or optic nerve pathology.

It is not unusual to see a mild eyelid reaction with edema and erythema. The conjunctiva is often mildly injected, and subconjunctival hemorrhage may be present. The cornea should be clear, but some superior edema is often present from the bending of the cornea during lens extraction. This edema generally resolves during the first postoperative week. The anterior chamber should be normal depth with mild to moderate cellular reaction. The pupil should be round and the iridectomy patent. A good red reflex should be present.

The postoperative course should be characterized by steady improvement of vision and comfort. Topical antibiotics and steroids are typically prescribed during the first postoperative weeks. The refraction generally becomes stable 6–12 weeks after intracapsular surgery, depending on the wound-closure technique employed. Because ICCE requires a larger incision, achieving a stable refraction usually takes longer after ICCE than after ECCE or phacoemulsification techniques, which require smaller incisions.

Types of Cataract Surgery: Extracapsular Cataract Extraction With Nucleus Expression

Indications

Extracapsular cataract extraction by nucleus expression was a major leap forward in modern cataract surgery. Selection of this technique depends on the instrumentation available, the surgeon's level of experience, and the density of the nucleus.

ECCE involves removal of the lens nucleus and cortex through an opening in the anterior capsule, leaving the capsular bag in place. This technique has a number of advantages over ICCE. Because it is performed through a smaller incision, it is generally

- less traumatic to the corneal endothelium
- associated with less induced astigmatism
- a more stable and secure wound

In addition, the posterior capsule is intact, which

- reduces the risk of intraoperative vitreous loss
- allows better anatomical position for IOL fixation
- reduces the incidence of CME, retinal detachment, and corneal edema
- reduces the iris and vitreous mobility that occurs with saccadic movements (endophthalmodonesis)
- provides a barrier restricting the exchange of some molecules between aqueous and vitreous
- reduces bacterial access to the vitreous cavity for endophthalmitis
- eliminates the short- and long-term complications associated with vitreous adherence to the iris, cornea, and incision

Subsequent secondary IOL implantation, filtration surgery, corneal transplantation, and wound repair are all technically easier and safer when an intact posterior capsule is present.

Contraindications

ECCE requires zonular integrity for the selective removal of the nucleus and cortical material. Therefore, when zonular support appears insufficient to allow safe removal of the cataract through extracapsular surgery, another cataract removal technique should be considered.

Instrumentation

A wide range of instruments is available for each step of ECCE, from opening the capsule to dissecting and extracting the lens nucleus, removing the lens cortex, and polishing the lens capsule. The *cystotome* is an instrument for anterior capsulotomy (the opening of the anterior capsule of the lens). Cystotomes can be fashioned from 25-gauge needles by bending the needle at its hub and where the beveled tip begins. Prefabricated cystotomes are also commercially available.

Blunt *cannulas* are used to irrigate and aspirate fluid within the eye during surgery; they come in various sizes and configurations. Cannulas may have an opening at the end of the tip or on the side of the tip to direct fluid flow. The gauge of the opening is determined by the instrument's intended function. Smaller ports develop high suction adhesion and are better for grasping and withdrawing material, whereas larger ports allow irrigation and aspiration of thicker substances such as viscoelastic agents and lens cortex. A coaxial, double-lumen cannula is commonly used for extracapsular surgery: one lumen irrigates balanced salt solution into the chamber while the second lumen aspirates lens material out of the chamber. Irrigation is gravity fed from a solution bottle; fluid flow is regulated with the adjustment of bottle height. The infusion may be constant, or the surgeon can employ a foot control connected to a pinch valve. Aspiration may simply involve a syringe connected to the cannula, or it may be part of an elaborate pump system controlled by a foot switch. Such automated systems are discussed further in Types of Cataract Surgery: Extracapsular Extraction by Phacoemulsification.

Procedure

Pupillary dilation is critical to the success of ECCE. Mydriatic/cycloplegic drops, administered preoperatively, effectively dilate the pupil, whereas topical nonsteroidal anti-inflammatory drops can help to maintain dilation during surgery.

Incision

Nucleus expression requires a midlimbal chord length of 8–12 mm, significantly smaller than the incision needed for ICCE. The initial incision usually consists of a limbal groove, fashioned with a round-tipped steel blade, sharp microknife, or diamond knife. Some surgeons prefer a slightly more posterior incision with anterior dissection creating a scleral flap or tunnel. These incisions are typically placed superiorly. A stab incision is made into the anterior chamber in preparation for an anterior capsulotomy, and the cystotome is inserted to begin the procedure. The anterior chamber depth can be stabilized by viscoelastic agents, air bubble, or continuous fluid irrigation.

Anterior capsulotomy

The main function of the anterior capsulotomy is to permit removal of the cataract while leaving behind the intact capsular bag, which provides stabilization for the IOL that will be implanted. There are many techniques for opening the anterior capsule. A sharp cystotome or bent needle may be used to make a series of connected punctures or small tears in a circle to create the "can-opener" capsulotomy (Fig 8-12A). Alternatively, a smooth capsulorrhexis may be created by making a puncture or small tear. The edge of this tear is then grasped with the cystotome tip or with a forceps and pulled around smoothly, removing a circular portion of anterior capsule (Fig 8-12B). This technique provides greater structural integrity for the lens capsule to maintain implant stability and centration. If a small capsulorrhexis is created and manual expression is planned, relaxing incisions are often made in the superior aspect of the capsulorrhexis to allow the nucleus adequate room to exit the capsule during expression. After the capsulotomy is completed, the wound is widened to allow safe passage of the nucleus through the incision. Anterior capsulotomy is discussed in greater detail in Types of Cataract Surgery: Extracapsular Extraction by Phacoemulsification.

Nucleus removal

Again, there are many different techniques for removal of the nucleus. Manual expression involves pressing on the inferior limbus to tip the superior pole of the nucleus up and out of the capsular bag. Additional counterpressure on the globe from an instrument holding the sclera posterior to the wound will express the nucleus from the chamber. The nucleus is removed from the eye by loosening and elevating it from the capsule with a hook or irrigating cannula, and then supporting it on a lens loop, spoon, or vectis that will slide or irrigate it out of the chamber. Alternatively, the nucleus may be fragmented within the eye using forceps or nucleus splitters to deliver it for removal in portions, through a smaller incision.

The wound is partially sutured to allow deepening of the chamber with irrigation. The lens cortex is then grasped and aspirated under direct visualization in the pupillary

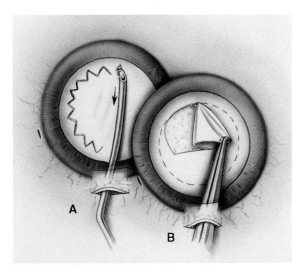

Figure 8-12 Anterior capsulotomy techniques. **A**, In the "can-opener" incision, punctures are made peripherally and pulled centrally so that the torn edges connect. Each puncture site has the potential for a radial tear if stressed. **B**, In the capsulorrhexis, tearing is begun within the area to be excised and finished from outside in. When stress lines in the free flap appear between forceps and the tear site, best control is maintained by regrasping the flap near the tear site. Positive pressure makes the tear travel peripherally; filling the anterior chamber with viscoelastic will counteract. *(Reproduced with permission from Johnson SH. Phacoemulsification.* Focal Points: Clinical Modules for Ophthalmologists. *San Francisco: American Academy of Ophthalmology; 1994, module 6. Illustration by Christine Gralapp.)*

space or withdrawn from the chamber using the aspiration cannula. The posterior capsule may be polished with an abrasive-tipped irrigation cannula, wiped with a silicone-lined "squeegee," or vacuumed clean using low aspiration to remove epithelial and cortical particles from the capsule surface.

IOL insertion

Prior to IOL insertion, the anterior chamber is usually filled with viscoelastic. Viscoelastics provide the most reliable anterior chamber maintenance along with protection of the corneal endothelium. (Viscoelastics are discussed in greater detail later in this chapter in Viscoelastics.)

A posterior chamber IOL may be inserted in the sulcus or in the capsular bag. Sulcus fixation usually requires an intraocular lens with a larger overall diameter (at least 12.5 mm) and a larger diameter optic (at least 6.0 mm), which is more forgiving in case of postoperative decentration.

If the surgeon wishes to insert the IOL into the capsular bag, viscoelastic is usually injected into the bag, with care being taken to fully separate the anterior capsular flap from the posterior capsule. Direct visualization of haptic insertion is critical. Smaller diameter IOLs may be used (less than 12.5 mm), as well as smaller diameter optics (5.0 mm round, 5.5 mm round, and 5.0 × 6.0 mm oval). However, recent studies have reported some problems with edge glare and other visual phenomena when smaller optic diameter IOLs were implanted, especially in patients who have significant mydriasis in the dark. (IOLs are discussed at length in Primary Intraocular Lens Implantation in Adults.)

Closure

The ECCE wound is typically closed with either multiple interrupted sutures of 10–0 nylon or with one long running suture (see Fig 8-9). Proper suture tension helps reduce postoperative astigmatism; loose sutures cause astigmatism perpendicular to the axis of the suture, whereas tight sutures create astigmatism in the axis of the suture.

Postoperative Course

As with ICCE, visual acuity on the first postoperative day should be consistent with the refractive state of the eye, the clarity of the cornea and media, and the visual potential of the retina and optic nerve. A mild eyelid reaction with edema and erythema may occur. The conjunctival flap may be injected and boggy, but it should not be elevated by fluid. The cornea may have some mild degree of edema. The anterior chamber should be of normal depth, and a mild cellular reaction is typical. The posterior capsule should be clear and intact, and the implant should be well positioned and stable. The red reflex should be strong and clear. IOP elevations may be associated with retained viscoelastic. Topical antibiotic and corticosteroid eyedrops are generally prescribed postoperatively.

The postoperative course should be characterized by steady improvement of vision and comfort, as the inflammatory reaction subsides during the first 2 weeks. The refraction is typically stable by the sixth to eighth postoperative week, and spectacles may then be prescribed. If a significant amount of postoperative astigmatism results along the axis of the sutures, the sutures can be selectively removed as guided by wound stability, keratometry, or corneal topography. This can be performed as soon as the sixth postoperative week.

Types of Cataract Surgery: Extracapsular Extraction by Phacoemulsification

Phacoemulsification is an extracapsular technique that differs from conventional ECCE with nuclear expression by the size of the incision required and the method of nucleus removal. This technique uses an ultrasonically driven tip to fragment the nucleus of the cataract and aspirate the lens. It results in a lower incidence of wound-related complications, faster healing, and more rapid visual rehabilitation than procedures that require larger incisions. This technique also creates a relatively closed system during both phacoemulsification and aspiration, thereby controlling anterior chamber depth and providing safeguards against positive vitreous pressure and choroidal hemorrhage.

Making the Transition

Most cataract surgeons skilled in extracapsular surgery choose to add phacoemulsification to their repertoire of surgical skills. In making the transition, the surgeon should alter technique slowly and cautiously. Phacoemulsification should be performed only after a training course that involves instruction on proper patient selection, specific surgical technique, and instrument parameters. A surgeon wishing to make a smooth transition to phacoemulsification should develop a personal plan to bridge the various differences in surgical technique. Observing an experienced phacoemulsification surgeon is helpful.

The surgeon should progress from cases in which the nucleus is moderately dense to those more difficult cases in which the nucleus is either very hard or very soft. In a similar fashion, progression can be made from a capsulotomy to a capsulorrhexis as the surgeon's level of comfort with the technique increases. Options for incisions include limbal, posterior scleral tunnel, and clear corneal. During the learning process, it is not advisable to change all of these parameters at once. If problems are encountered in the process, the surgeon may convert to standard ECCE at any time during the surgery.

Patient Selection

Ideally, the first patient should be a cooperative individual who can lie still a long time without shortness of breath or agitation. The surgeon's first phacoemulsification will probably take longer than the familiar ECCE. A patient whose iris dilates widely is preferable. Other ideal characteristics include a clear cornea without opacities to ensure intraoperative visualization and the absence of corneal guttatae, which increase the risk of postoperative corneal edema. Eyes with a normal axial length of 22–24 mm are preferred. Highly myopic eyes can have significant scleral thinning, reduced scleral rigidity, and very deep anterior chambers. Patients with high hyperopia have small eyes and shallower anterior chambers, making surgery more difficult technically.

The surgeon should pay careful attention to the patient's orbital anatomy. Shallow orbits allow better surgical exposure than deep ones. With a deep orbit, the phacoemulsification handpiece must be held in a more vertical orientation, and the eye must be rotated downward to allow the instrument to enter through the superior wound. Visualization and manipulation of the handpiece become more awkward. Ultimately, these deep-set eyes are much more easily and safely approached with a temporal clear corneal incision.

The first cases should involve a moderately dense nucleus. In general, patient age and the degree of brunescence correlate well with density of the nucleus. If the patient is older than 75 years, the surgeon should anticipate that the nucleus will be relatively hard. The surgeon may wish to avoid eyes with exfoliation syndrome because the zonular fibers and capsule in these cases are weak, and the pupils may not dilate well. Patients with subluxated or dislocated lenses should also be avoided.

Instrumentation

The instruments used in phacoemulsification involve both ultrasonics and fluid dynamics. With the newer generation of phacoemulsification machines, it is now possible to vary all the parameters at each stage of the procedure. The Phacoemulsification Glossary defines some of the most important terms and concepts of ultrasonics and fluidics. See Procedure, Instrument Settings for Phacoemulsification later in this section for specific instrument settings for nuclear sculpting, emulsification, and aspiration.

Phacoemulsification Glossary

Ultrasonics Terminology

Cavitation The formation of vacuoles in a liquid by a swiftly moving solid body, such as the ultrasonic tip. The collapse of the vacuoles releases energy that vaporizes and crushes lens material.

Chatter To cut unevenly with rapidly intermittent vibration. Chatter occurs when the ultrasonic stroke overcomes the vacuum, or "holding power." This causes the nuclear fragments to be repelled by the ultrasonic tip until the vacuum reaches high enough levels to neutralize the ultrasonic tip's repulsive energy. Chatter inhibits followability (defined under Fluidics Terminology).

Frequency In phacoemulsification, how fast the phaco needle moves back and forth. The frequency of current ultrasonic handpieces is between 27,000 and 60,000 strokes per second.

Load In ultrasonics, occurs when the ultrasonic tip encounters nuclear material. Load requires that the system and the ultrasonic tip maintain constant stroke length or power. Because load is constantly changing, the system must be able to adapt to the changing conditions. If the system cannot, then the cutting efficiency will be compromised.

Piezoelectric A type of transducer used in ultrasonic handpieces that transforms electrical energy into mechanical energy. Linear motion is generated when a tuned, highly refined crystal is deformed by the electrical energy supplied by the console.

Power The ability of the phaco needle to vibrate and cavitate the adjacent lens material. Power is referred to by a percentage on the instrument panel of most phacoemulsification machines. This percentage of power is proportional to the stroke length.

Stroke A sudden action or process producing an impact. This impact is measured by the magnitude of tip movement, which occurs at an ultrasonic frequency between 27,000 Hz and 60,000 Hz. Stroke length at 100% power varies between the various manufacturers from 2–4 mils (0.002–0.004 in.).

Tuning The method used to match the optimum driving frequency of the ultrasonic board within the console with the operating frequency of the phacoemulsification handpiece.

Ultrasonic Frequencies above the range of human audibility, or above 20,000 vibrations per second. In phacoemulsification, the term *ultrasonic* is used because the phaco needle moves back and forth in excess of 20,000 times per second.

Fluidics Terminology

Aspiration The withdrawal of fluid from the eye.

Aspiration flow rate The rate at which fluid is removed from the eye. Aspiration flow rate generates the force that attracts material to the distal end of the phaco handpiece. It is one of the primary factors that determines how fast the fluidic system responds. Other factors are compliance, venting, and tubing size.

Followability The ability of a fluidic system to attract and hold nuclear or cortical material on the distal end of an ultrasonic or irrigation/aspiration handpiece. Followability depends on pressure gradient/difference between the IOP and aspiration port. It can also be negatively affected by the forward acoustical wave of a vibrating ultrasonic tip.

Occlusion An obstruction of the aspiration port or aspiration tubing. Occlusion usually occurs when nuclear or cortical material is being aspirated from the eye. Occlusion is necessary to create vacuum.

Rise time The rate at which vacuum builds once the aspiration port has been occluded. Rise time is directly related to the aspiration flow rate, which is related to the pump speed. The faster the aspiration flow rate (or pump speed), the faster the rise time.

Surge A phenomenon that usually occurs when vacuum has built up because of an occlusion and the occlusion is suddenly broken, leading to the fluid in the higher-pressure (positive) anterior chamber tending to rush into the lower-pressure (negative) phaco tip. If the negative surge exceeds the inflow capability of the irrigation line, anterior chamber depth fluctuations may occur.

Vacuum The suction force exerted on the fluid in the aspiration line of the eye. Vacuum, or negative pressure, is the holding force for material that has occluded the aspiration port. The higher the vacuum, the greater the holding force. Vacuum is measured in millimeters of mercury (mm Hg) or inches of water.

Venting Also known as "exposing to the air," the process whereby negative pressure or vacuum is equalized to atmospheric levels to minimize surge.

Ultrasound

The phaco handpiece contains a piezoelectric crystal that vibrates at a frequency of 27,000–60,000 Hz. The vibration is transmitted along the handpiece to the phaco tip, where the primary oscillation is axial. There are several varieties of tips, varied according to the angle of the tip and the size of the lumen. Phaco tips are available in 0°, 15°, 30°, 45°, 60°, and combined 30/60° (turbo) beveled tips (Fig 8-13). In general, the surgeon chooses the bevel angle of the phaco tip based on personal preference but with the

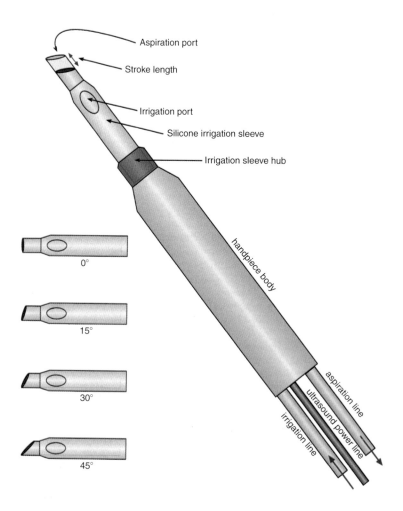

Figure 8-13 Parts of a phaco handpiece; smaller drawings depict the different tip bevels available. *(Reprinted with permission from Seibel BS.* Phacodynamics: Mastering the Tools and Techniques of Phacoemulsification Surgery. *3rd ed. Thorofare, NJ: Slack; 1999.)*

understanding that lower-angle beveled tips are better for engaging nuclear material, whereas steeper tip bevels are better for cutting nuclear material. A 0° tip has the minimum possible surface area for its aspiration port. The area is the needle's internal diameter. Tips with a greater bevel have an oval-shaped port with a larger surface area. Because pressure is defined as force per unit area, the tips with the greater surface area can generate greater gripping force (Fig 8-14).

Most phaco tips are 18 gauge, but some are as small as 23 gauge. The smaller-bore tips allow for higher and more efficient vacuum, thus creating a better purchase on the nuclear material. Phaco tips may be straight or angled. Angled tips allow for more efficient cavitation and more effective cutting of hard nuclei. The primary direction of ultrasonic oscillation is axial, and cavitation is usually limited to the area in front of the ring of

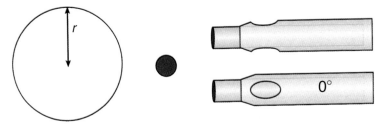

Holding force per 100 mm Hg = .0019 lb

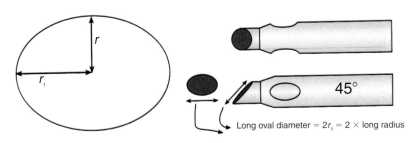

Holding force per 100 mm Hg = .0027 lb

Figure 8-14 Drawing depicts the relationship between the phaco tip bevel and holding force. *(Reprinted with permission from Seibel BS.* Phacodynamics: Mastering the Tools and Techniques of Phacoemulsification Surgery. *3rd ed. Thorofare, NJ: Slack; 1999.)*

metal at the front of the needle (Fig 8-15). Cavitation can be enhanced by changes in the needle shape. For example, the distal bend in the angled Kelman tip adds a nonaxial vibration to the primary oscillation. The nonaxial vibration augments the axial vibration and produces an elliptical motion at the cutting tip, which increases the total cavitation at the tip and enhances the mechanical breakdown of nuclear material.

Emulsification and removal of the nuclear material require careful coordination of cutting, ultrasonic fragmentation, and aspiration. The sharp tip mechanically disrupts the tissue; the vibration causes cavitation of the lens material close to the tip; and aspiration through the port removes the mechanically disrupted and cavitated tissue through the needle. The process of needle movement and cavitation pushes lens material away from the needle port, while aspiration constantly draws the material toward the port of the probe. Understanding this interrelationship is important for grasping the dynamics of phacoemulsification.

Phacoemulsification continues to evolve through advances in technology and technique. Early phacoemulsification machines vibrated at a constant power with constant aspiration. Earlier techniques, therefore, required very rapid sculpting of the nucleus, using steeply beveled tips. Minimal attention was given to the aspiration and vacuum modes.

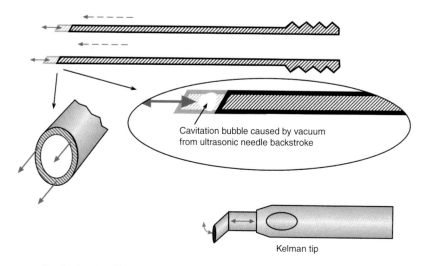

Cavitation bubble caused by vacuum
from ultrasonic needle backstroke

Kelman tip

Figure 8-15 Cavitation is affected by the angle of the phaco tip as well as by different needle shapes. *(Reprinted with permission from Seibel BS. Phacodynamics: Mastering the Tools and Techniques of Phacoemulsification Surgery. 3rd ed. Thorofare, NJ: Slack; 1999.)*

However, since the introduction of variable-power phacoemulsification, the trend has been to emphasize the active control of aspiration and vacuum, while using the phacoemulsification power secondarily. This fundamental difference has led to the use of lower phacoemulsification power and has given more control over the phacoemulsification process. Ideally, the surgeon uses only enough phacoemulsification power to fragment and aspirate the nuclear material.

Newer technologies include the WhiteStar system (Advanced Medical Optics, Santa Ana, CA), which uses high-rate microbursts of phacoemulsification energy that result in much lower heat buildup at the phaco tip. Other systems also offer burst or pulse mode to decrease heat buildup, lower total phacoemulsification energy, and improve followability.

Irrigation

The fluid dynamics of phacoemulsification require constant irrigation through the irrigation sleeve around the ultrasound tip, with some egress of fluid across the wound. Constant irrigation maintains anterior chamber depth and cools the phaco probe, preventing heat buildup with adjacent tissue damage. Use of chilled irrigation fluid has been advocated by some, who claim that the cold fluid cools the probe more effectively, constricts blood vessels, maintains corneal clarity better, and may even stabilize the blood-aqueous barrier.

Aspiration

The aspiration system of phacoemulsification machines varies according to pump design. The 3 types of pumps are peristaltic, diaphragm, and Venturi. All 3 types are based on the principle of creating vacuum by means of occlusion. Thus, if the aspiration port is not occluded, vacuum cannot be generated.

The *peristaltic pump* consists of a set of rollers that move along flexible tubing, forcing fluid through the tubing and creating a relative vacuum at the aspiration port of the phaco tip (Fig 8-16). Vacuum response time with this type of pump is relatively rapid; linear control is achieved by increasing the speed of the rollers.

A *diaphragm pump* consists of a flexible diaphragm overlying a fluid chamber with 1-way valves at the inlet and outlet. The diaphragm moves out, creating a relative vacuum in the chamber that shuts the exit valve, causing the fluid to flow into the chamber. The diaphragm then moves in, which increases the pressure in the chamber and closes the intake valve while opening the exit valve (Fig 8-17). This type of pump system produces a slower rise in vacuum. With continued occlusion of the aspiration port, however, the vacuum will continue to increase in an exponential manner.

The *Venturi pump* creates a vacuum based on the Venturi principle: a flow of gas or fluid across a port creates a vacuum proportional to the rate of flow of the gas (Fig 8-18). This system produces a rapid, linear rise in vacuum and allows for instantaneous venting to the atmosphere that immediately stops the flow through the port.

In general, all of these pumps are effective. The vacuum rise time (the amount of time required to reach a given level of vacuum) varies among the different pump designs (Fig 8-19). The surgeon should consider the rise time of the instrument being used in

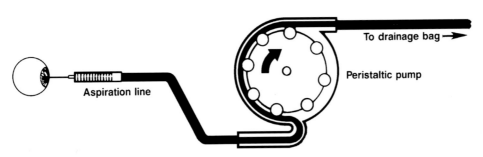

Figure 8-16 The peristaltic pump. *(Redrawn with permission from* Practical Phacoemulsification: Proceedings of the Third Annual Workshop. *Montreal, Quebec: Medicopea International, Inc; 1991:43–48.)*

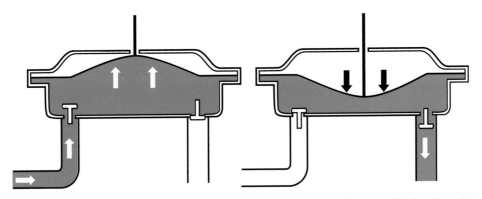

Figure 8-17 The diaphragm pump. *(Redrawn with permission from* Practical Phacoemulsification: Proceedings of the Third Annual Workshop. *Montreal, Quebec: Medicopea International, Inc; 1991:43–48.)*

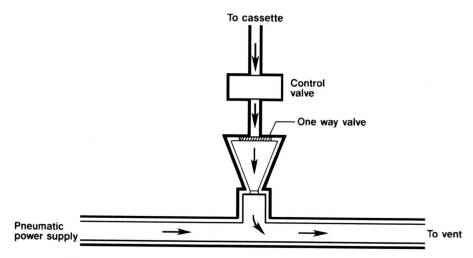

Figure 8-18 The Venturi pump. *(Redrawn with permission from* Practical Phacoemulsification: Proceedings of the Third Annual Workshop. *Montreal, Quebec: Medicopea International, Inc; 1991:43–48.)*

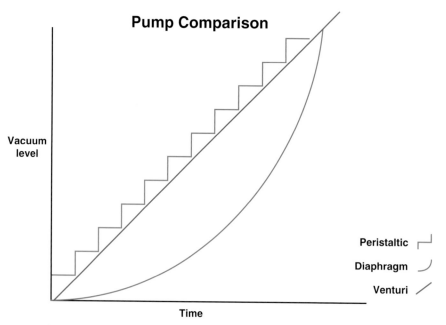

Figure 8-19 Comparison of vacuum rise times in the peristaltic, diaphragm, and Venturi pumps. *(Redrawn with permission from* Practical Phacoemulsification: Proceedings of the Third Annual Workshop. *Montreal, Quebec: Medicopea International, Inc; 1991:43–48.)*

planning a specific technique. The diaphragm pump has a slow rise time, with pressure building in an exponential fashion after occlusion of the port. The peristaltic pump has a stepwise rise in pressure after occlusion of the port. The Venturi pump, which has a smoother rise in pressure after occlusion of the port, creates an instantaneous vacuum. Furthermore, the vacuum rise time is inversely proportional to the aspiration flow rate. The faster the flow rate, the shorter the rise time will be. Conversely, for example, as the aspiration flow rate is decreased by half, from 40 to 20 cc/minute, the vacuum rise time is doubled, from 1 to 2 seconds (Fig 8-20). An additional halving of the flow rate from 20 to 10 cc/minute is also associated with a doubling of the rise time from 2 to 4 seconds.

Specific instrument settings and the nuances of the interaction of aspiration, vacuum, and power are discussed in detail later in this section in Procedure, Instrument Settings for Phacoemulsification.

Procedure

Patient preparation

As with conventional ECCE, pupillary dilation with mydriatic/cycloplegic drops is recommended. Pupil-stretching techniques or special iris retractors can be used to open miotic pupils unresponsive to pharmacologic dilation (see Ocular Conditions, Glaucoma, Complications of Cataract Surgery in the Glaucoma Patient in Chapter 10).

Exposure of the globe

The eyelids are usually held apart during surgery with a lid speculum, although some surgeons prefer sterile adhesive strips or sutures to keep the lids apart. In selecting an eyelid speculum, the surgeon must take into account the size and location of the handpiece as it moves within the surgical field.

Incisions

Scleral tunnel incision   The scleral tunnel incision with an internal corneal lip is commonly used by cataract surgeons. This incision gives the phacoemulsification surgeon an excellent degree of control during the procedure, and it also allows for conversion to conventional ECCE if necessary. It entails a 2-planed incision that begins in the sclera to prevent induced postoperative astigmatism and ends in the clear peripheral cornea (distal to the iris root) to prevent iris prolapse (Fig 8-21).

A bridle suture may be placed to help position the globe for surgery. The bridle suture is especially helpful to the beginning phacoemulsification surgeon for stabilizing the globe and exposing the bulbar conjunctiva to create a conjunctival flap. Many experienced surgeons ultimately dispense with the superior rectus bridle suture; doing so may reduce the risk of postoperative ptosis.

The surgeon then creates a conjunctival flap. Although a limbal-based conjunctival flap can be used, a fornix-based flap is preferable because it affords an unobstructed view of the sclera and limbus without manipulation. After creating the conjunctival flap, the surgeon clears the overlying Tenon's capsule from the sclera and applies light bipolar cautery to achieve hemostasis. (Excessive cautery is to be avoided, as it may cause scleral shrinkage and postoperative astigmatism.) The initial scleral incision should be perpen-

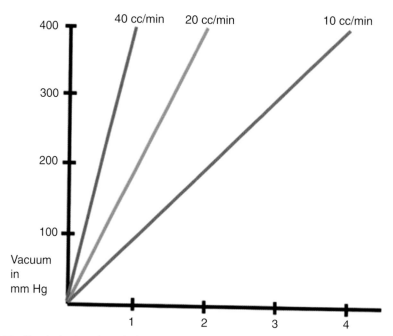

400

40 cc/min   20 cc/min   10 cc/min

300

200

100

Vacuum
in
mm Hg

1   2   3   4

Figure 8-20 Graph depicts the relationship between aspiration flow rate and vacuum rise time. *(Reprinted with permission from Seibel BS.* Phacodynamics: Mastering the Tools and Techniques of Phacoemulsification Surgery. *3rd ed. Thorofare, NJ: Slack; 1999.)*

dicular to the scleral surface at a depth of about 0.3 mm and placed 1.0–3.0 mm posterior to the surgical limbus. The initial incision length should be 2.75–7.0 mm, depending on the style of IOL to be implanted. Foldable IOLs can be inserted through 2.75–4.0-mm incisions, whereas all PMMA IOLs require openings slightly larger than the diameter of the optic. Internal incision size should be at least as large as the external dimension. The scleral incision is usually linear (tangential to the limbus), but it may be curvilinear (following the limbus or following the curve opposite the limbus) or chevron-shaped (Fig 8-22).

The surgeon then uses a blade to enter the scleral groove at a chosen depth and dissects anteriorly, parallel to the corneal-scleral surface and into clear cornea, developing a tunnel incision (see Fig 8-21). The tunnel incision is carried forward, just anterior to the vascular arcade. If the scleral groove is entered too deeply, the scleral flap will be very thick and the blade may penetrate the anterior chamber earlier than anticipated, closer to the vascular iris root. If the scleral groove is entered superficially, the scleral flap will be very thin and prone to tears or buttonholes. Either metal or diamond knives may be used for fashioning the scleral tunnel, but beginning surgeons may benefit from the added resistance and the tactile feedback provided by a metal blade.

A small paracentesis is then placed approximately 2 or 3 clock-hours away from the scleral tunnel to provide an entry site for the second instrument used to manipulate the lens in most 2-handed techniques. Injecting viscoelastic through the paracentesis at this stage helps to maintain the IOP and anterior chamber depth, thereby making the sub-

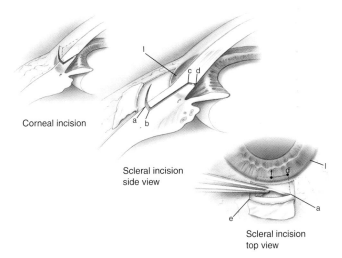

Corneal incision

Scleral incision
side view

Scleral incision
top view

Figure 8-21 Two types of phacoemulsification incisions. Detail for scleral incision, side view: *a to b*: Initial groove is 1/3–1/2 of scleral depth; if groove is too deep, bleeding may increase and entry into anterior chamber is likely to be too posterior, causing iris prolapse. *a to l*: Incision is traditionally 2–3 mm posterior to limbus. *b to c*: Tunnel is traditionally dissected past vascular arcade; if too long, ultrasound tip mobility is restricted and corneal striae decrease visibility. *c to d*: Short third plane is made by changing angle of blade prior to entering anterior chamber. In scleral incision, top view: *e to a*: Length of incision is determined by size of IOL. *f to d*: Initial opening into anterior chamber is usually 3.0–3.25 mm; after phacoemulsification, it is fully opened for IOL insertion. If opening is too small, irrigation flow is decreased, chamber tends to shallow, and heat buildup may cause burn. If opening is too large, excessive fluid egress causes chamber shallowing and iris may prolapse. *(Reproduced with permission from Johnson SH. Phacoemulsification. Focal Points: Clinical Modules for Ophthalmologists. San Francisco: American Academy of Ophthalmology; 1994, module 6. Illustration by Christine Gralapp.)*

sequent keratome entry into the anterior chamber easier and safer. The surgeon uses a keratome sized to match the phaco tip width to enter the anterior chamber beneath the scleral flap. The keratome is inserted in the tunnel until it reaches the clear cornea beyond the vascular arcade. The heel of the keratome is elevated and the tip of the keratome is pointed posteriorly, aiming toward the center of the lens and creating a dimple in the peripheral cornea. The keratome is then slowly advanced in this posterior direction, creating an internal corneal lip as it enters the anterior chamber. The stepped incision is used in order to create a valve that allows the wound to be self-sealing once the anterior chamber is re-formed. Some surgeons prefer to fill the anterior chamber with viscoelastic after the keratome entry. If the scleral tunnel is too long, it can cause difficulties in manipulating the phaco tip within the anterior chamber. If the tunnel incision extends too far anteriorly in clear cornea, visibility can be reduced by corneal striae and distortion as the phaco tip is being manipulated.

Clear corneal incision Many surgeons now prefer to perform phacoemulsification and insert a foldable IOL through a clear corneal incision at the temporal limbus, often with the use of topical anesthesia. Advocates of this approach cite the speed of the operation

124 • Lens and Cataract

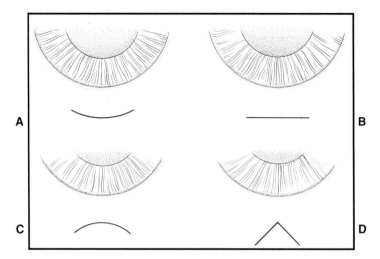

Figure 8-22 External scleral grooves can be made in various configurations, including posterior and parallel to the limbus **(A)**; tangential to the limbus **(B)**; curving away from the limbus: the "frown" incision **(C)**; or chevron-shaped **(D)**. *(Reproduced with permission from Masket S. Cataract incision and closure. Focal Points: Clinical Modules for Ophthalmologists. San Francisco: American Academy of Ophthalmology; 1995, module 3. Illustration by Christine Gralapp.)*

and the rapid visual rehabilitation. The initial corneal incision is made just large enough to accommodate the phaco tip in order to maintain a deep anterior chamber that does not fluctuate during phacoemulsification. The wound may need to be enlarged slightly, in the range of 2.7–4.0 mm, to insert the foldable IOL, depending on the IOL and insertion technology used.

Globe stabilization is important in clear corneal incisions, especially if performed under topical anesthesia. Fixation rings, 0.12 forceps, and even muscle hooks supplying counterpressure can be used to stabilize the globe as the incisions are made. The paracentesis is made first, followed by injection of intracameral, nonpreserved lidocaine, if desired. Viscoelastic is injected through the paracentesis to stabilize the anterior chamber depth and maintain the IOP for the subsequent keratome entry.

One approach for the clear corneal incision is a *multiplanar incision* using a vertical corneal groove (Fig 8-23). In the technique introduced by Langerman, a diamond or metal knife is used to create a 0.3-mm-deep groove perpendicular to the corneal surface. Another blade is inserted in the groove, and its tip is then directed tangential to the corneal surface, thereby creating a 2.0-mm tunnel through the clear cornea into the anterior chamber. This biplanar wound architecture is usually watertight. A variation on this biplanar incision involves making a deeper vertical groove and creating a hinge.

A more popular approach is the *beveled, biplanar, self-sealing incision,* as advocated by Shimuzu and Fine. A beveled 3-mm diamond blade is flattened against the eye, and the tip is used to enter the cornea just anterior to the vascular arcade. The blade is advanced tangentially to the corneal surface until the shoulders of the blade are fully buried in the stroma. The point of the blade is then redirected posteriorly so that the point and the rest of the blade enter the anterior chamber parallel to the iris. This

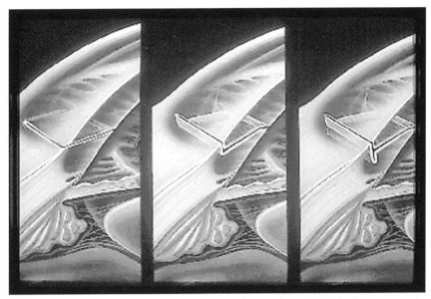

Figure 8-23 Architecture of clear corneal incisions. Single plane *(left)*, shallow groove *(center)*, and deep groove *(right)*. *(Reprinted with permission from Fine IH.* Clear Corneal Lens Surgery. *Thorofare, NJ: Slack; 1999.)*

technique ideally creates a 3 × 2-mm corneal wound that is watertight. Disposable steel blades can also be used to create these incisions. Newer beveled, trapezoidal diamond blades have been developed for self-sealing clear corneal incisions. Such blades can be advanced in one motion and in one plane, from clear cornea into the anterior chamber (Fig 8-24). The blade is oriented parallel to the iris (0°), and the tip is placed at the start of the clear cornea, just anterior to the vascular arcades. The blade is tilted up and the heel down so that the blade is angled 10° from the iris plane and then advanced into the anterior chamber in one smooth, continuous motion. Regardless of which type of clear corneal incision is used, the goal is to keep the incision just large enough to accommodate the folded IOL with its inserter, generally 2.7–4.0 mm. Newer technologies under development will, in the near future, permit lens removal and IOL insertion through a 1.2-mm incision.

After the cataract is removed and the IOL has been inserted, the viscoelastic is removed, the anterior chamber is re-formed with sterile balanced salt solution via the paracentesis site, and the wound is examined for leakage. If the wound leaks, both sides of the corneal tunnel incision can be hydrated with sterile balanced salt solution injected through a syringe with a blunt 25- to 26-gauge irrigating tip. Hydration of the corneal incision causes temporary stromal swelling and increases the wound apposition between the roof and the floor of the tunnel, thereby eliminating any leakage. If this maneuver fails to stop the leak, a single radial 10–0 nylon suture in the center of the incision with a buried knot will usually suffice.

Ernest PH, Neuhann T. Posterior limbal incision. *J Cataract Refract Surg.* 1996;22:78–84.

Fine IH. Corneal tunnel incision with a temporal approach. In: Fine IH, Fichman RA, Grabow

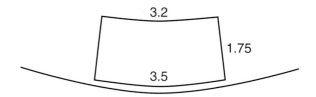

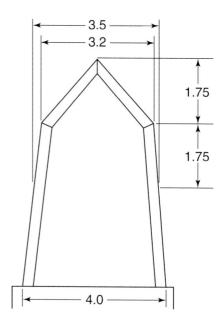

Figure 8-24 *Below,* Dimensions and shape of a beveled, trapezoidal diamond blade used in clear corneal incisions and *(above)* contour of the incision made with this knife. *(Reprinted with permission from Fine IH, Fichman RA, Grabow HB. Clear-Corneal Cataract Surgery and Topical Anesthesia. Thorofare, NJ: Slack; 1993.)*

HB, eds. *Clear-Corneal Cataract Surgery and Topical Anesthesia.* Thorofare, NJ: Slack; 1993:50–51.

Langerman DW. Architectural design of a self-sealing corneal tunnel, single-hinge incision. *J Cataract Refract Surg.* 1994;20:84–88.

Anterior capsulotomy

Although a can-opener capsulotomy can be used with phacoemulsification, *continuous-tear circular capsulorrhexis* provides a more stable, smoother edge to the anterior capsular opening that resists radial tears and is definitely the preferred technique. The majority of cataract surgeons prefer an opening 0.5 mm smaller than the optic so the edge of the optic is completely covered. The purported benefits of this geometry are decreased capsular opacification and better IOL centration. Use of a small capsulorrhexis usually requires splitting the nucleus *(nucleofractis),* rather than removing it as a whole in the iris plane.

The surgeon begins an anterior capsulorrhexis with a central linear cut in the anterior capsule, using a cystotome needle (see Figure 8-12B). At the end of the linear cut, the needle is either pushed or pulled in the direction of the desired tear, allowing the anterior capsule to fold over upon itself. The surgeon then engages the free edge of the anterior capsule with either forceps or the capsulotomy needle, and the flap is carried around in a circular manner as the surgeon directs the tension toward the center of the lens. For maximum control, frequent regrasping of the flap near the tear is helpful. If a radial tear extends toward the equator during capsulorrhexis, the surgeon may need to convert to a can-opener capsulotomy technique. Radial extension of the capsulotomy may occur in the setting of forward displacement of the lens with shallowing of the anterior chamber or anterior traction on the capsular flap.

If the capsulorrhexis tear starts to extend too far peripherally, the flap can sometimes be salvaged and the tear brought more centrally. First, the surgeon should check for positive vitreous pressure associated with forward displacement of the lens. This may be caused by the capsulotomy instrument, the surgeon's fingers, or the lid speculum pressing against the globe; and it can be corrected. Refilling the anterior chamber with viscoelastic, and/or inserting a second instrument (such as an iris spatula) through the paracentesis to press posteriorly on the lens may help reduce forward displacement of the lens and allow for redirection of the capsular tear. Using the bent cystotome needle to redirect the tear centrally may also be helpful, as this instrument causes minimal wound distortion when inserted in the eye, and it can create sharp changes in the direction of the tear over very short distances. Often, several of these just-described maneuvers need to be employed in order to redirect and salvage the capsulorrhexis.

Hydrodissection

Following capsulorrhexis, gentle injection of irrigating fluid is performed to separate the peripheral cortex from the underlying capsule. In addition to loosening the lens nucleus/cortex complex, this procedure facilitates nuclear rotation during phacoemulsification and hydrates the peripheral cortex, making it easier to aspirate after nucleus removal. The surgeon places a bent, blunt-tipped 25- to 30-gauge needle attached to a 3-cc syringe under the anterior capsular flap. While the capsular flap is gently lifted, balanced salt solution is injected to hydrodissect the posterior cortical lamellae from the capsule. Gentle irrigation should continue until the surgeon sees a wave of fluid moving across the red reflex zone. Gentle posterior pressure centrally on the nucleus will express the posterior fluid and complete the hydrodissection. If the nucleus is displaced into the anterior chamber, it can be reposited into the posterior chamber with viscoelastic and gentle pressure. Hydrodissection is riskier after a can-opener capsulotomy and may result in significant radial tears that can extend posteriorly and threaten the posterior capsular integrity.

Hydrodelineation

Some surgeons also inject balanced salt solution into the substance of the nucleus to hydrodelineate, or separate, the various layers of the nucleus. This technique separates the harder endonucleus from the softer, outer epinucleus, which can remain behind to act as a cushion to protect the underlying posterior capsule from inadvertent trauma during nucleus removal.

Location of phacoemulsification

The nucleus may be emulsified at various locations within the eye, including the anterior chamber, iris plane, and posterior chamber. The location chosen for emulsification will determine which techniques are employed for nucleus management.

Anterior chamber When the technique of phacoemulsification was first developed, the anterior chamber was the preferred location for it. Various maneuvers evolved to prolapse the nucleus into the anterior chamber, after which the lens could be manipulated with relative ease and excellent visualization. Loss of pupillary dilation is less of a problem in this location, and the risk of posterior capsule damage or rupture is minimized because of the distance between the lens and capsule. However, the risk of corneal endothelial trauma is significant because of the proximity of the phaco needle to the endothelium. This technique is now used less frequently; it is used if the posterior capsule has ruptured and the surgeon must prevent the nucleus from subluxating into the vitreous or the patient has high myopia with a very deep anterior chamber.

Iris plane A later development was to perform the phacoemulsification at the iris plane. In this location, the superior pole of the nucleus was prolapsed anteriorly and emulsification occurred halfway between the corneal endothelium and the posterior capsule, thereby reducing the risk of damage to either structure. Once prolapsed, the nucleus could be manipulated with less stress on the posterior capsule and zonular fibers. In patients with small pupils, this technique permits placement of the nucleus within the pupil, thus maintaining visualization and allowing for safe emulsification.

The iris plane location is often desirable for the beginning phacoemulsification surgeon and in cases with small pupils or compromised capsular or zonular integrity. The disadvantages of this technique include the difficulty in prolapsing the nucleus and potential damage to the corneal endothelium if the superior pole of the nucleus is emulsified too close to the cornea.

Posterior chamber The posterior chamber is now considered the preferred location for phacoemulsification. Nucleus manipulation in this location requires capsulorrhexis, hydrodissection, and one of several techniques of nuclear splitting. The advantages of posterior chamber phacoemulsification are the reduced risk of corneal endothelial trauma and the ability to minimize the size of the capsulorrhexis opening, which is useful with suboptimal dilation. The disadvantages include the need to emulsify close to the posterior capsule, the greater stress placed on the posterior capsule and zonular fibers when the nucleus is being manipulated, the technical difficulty in small-pupil cases, and the need to employ more sophisticated methods of nuclear splitting.

Supracapsular A more recent innovation is the supracapsular phacoemulsification. This technique is described in greater detail later in Procedure, Nuclear-splitting Techniques. The essence of this technique is prolapsing the nucleus through the capsulorrhexis during hydrodissection and then replacing the nucleus into the posterior chamber on top of the capsular bag. This approach theoretically reduces the stress on the zonules during nucleus manipulation, can be used in small-pupil cases, and keeps the phaco tip and energy away from the corneal endothelium above and the posterior capsule below.

Endolenticular An endolenticular approach has been developed that uses a very small opening (3 mm) in the anterior capsule through which the entire emulsification process occurs. The advantages of this process, which is virtually confined to the capsular bag, include maximum endothelial protection and the future possibility of injecting synthetic lens material into an almost intact capsular bag. In addition to the overall technical difficulty, however, the disadvantages include the increased risk of posterior capsular rupture during both hydrodissection and emulsification and the need to enlarge the capsulorrhexis prior to IOL implantation.

Whole-nucleus removal

The nucleus can be emulsified as a whole in either the iris plane or the posterior chamber. The emulsification can be performed using either a 1-handed or 2-handed technique. If an iris plane approach is desired, a can-opener capsulotomy, pear-shaped capsulorrhexis, or generous circular capsulotomy is preferred. Following central nuclear sculpting and creation of a circular or D-shaped nuclear bowl (Fig 8-25), a 2-handed technique is used to prolapse the superior pole of the nucleus into the iris plane. The second instrument (eg, iris spatula or lens manipulator), inserted through the paracentesis, is used to push inferiorly on the nuclear bowl, while the phaco handpiece is used to spear the exposed superior pole of the nucleus (Fig 8-26). Irrigation through the phaco handpiece now creates a fluid wave that helps separate the posterior cortex from the underlying capsule. Using this classic 2-handed technique, the surgeon then lifts and exposes the superior pole of the nucleus and emulsifies the rim from the 11 o'clock to 1 o'clock positions. The nucleus is then rotated, continually exposing another segment of the rim for emulsification. The remaining nuclear plate is then carefully elevated off the posterior capsule and emulsified.

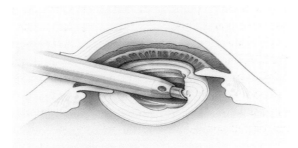

Figure 8-25 Central sculpting of the nucleus when managed as a whole. If the iris plane approach is used, the nucleus is sculpted to ½–⅔ its depth, leaving an inferior ledge; if the posterior chamber approach is used, the nucleus is sculpted deep centrally and thinned inferiorly to weaken the remaining lens material. *(Reproduced with permission from Johnson SH. Phacoemulsification. Focal Points: Clinical Modules for Ophthalmologists. San Francisco: American Academy of Ophthalmology; 1994, module 6. Illustration by Christine Gralapp.)*

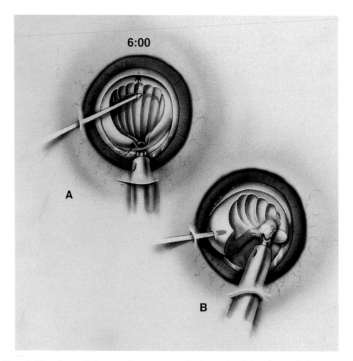

Figure 8-26 Emulsification of the nucleus as a whole at the iris plane, following central sculpting. **A,** Lens is subluxed by pushing the spatula against the ledge to move the lens toward 6 o'clock, leaving the anterior-posterior plane of the spatula unchanged. The anterior chamber is shallowed by stopping irrigation, allowing the superior lens equator to present anteriorly as the lens rotates around the stable spatula. The ultrasound tip is partially withdrawn to catch the posterior surface of the superior lens equator and help lift the lens. **B,** Nucleus is stabilized by sticking it with the spatula, and the ultrasound tip debulks the lens by quadrants. Both instruments are used to rotate the lens counterclockwise as the process continues. *(Reproduced with permission from Johnson SH. Phacoemulsification. Focal Points: Clinical Modules for Ophthalmologists. San Francisco: American Academy of Ophthalmology; 1994, module 6. Illustration by Christine Gralapp.)*

It is possible for the whole-nucleus emulsification to be performed in the capsular bag after adequate hydrodissection. This technique was refined and popularized by Fine and described as "chip and flip."

Chip and flip technique With a small anterior capsulorrhexis, the surgeon may use a *chip and flip technique.* After adequate hydrodissection and hydrodelineation, the surgeon removes the central core of the nucleus by sculpting, creating a nuclear bowl. The second instrument, a nucleus rotator, is inserted through the paracentesis, and the nucleus is pushed toward the incision. The phaco tip is then used to remove the rim of the inner nuclear bowl from the opposite nuclear rim. The nucleus is rotated clockwise, and another clock hour of rim is emulsified. By displacing the nucleus toward the incision, the surgeon pulls the part of the nucleus being emulsified away from the capsular fornix and out from under the iris, thereby improving visualization and protecting the underlying capsule. This process is repeated until the entire rim of inner nuclear bowl is removed, and the posterior nuclear chip remains.

The remaining nuclear chip is elevated with the second instrument and emulsified in the center of the capsular bag, with the soft epinuclear bowl acting as a cushion to protect the underlying capsule. (*Epinucleus* is a clinical term used to describe the outermost part of the nucleus or the innermost part of the cortex.) The second instrument is then used to push the epinuclear bowl away from the incision, allowing the soft epinuclear rim to curl over on itself, up toward the incision, until the entire epinuclear bowl has tumbled or flipped. This procedure is facilitated by aspirating the rim with the phaco tip at 6 o'clock and pulling superiorly. The flipped epinucleus is now easily and safely removed with either aspiration alone or low-power emulsification.

Nucleus-splitting techniques

The more recent and increasingly popular approach of nucleus splitting usually requires 2 instruments to subdivide the nucleus prior to its emulsification. Most frequently with these techniques, the nucleus is divided into the harder, central endonucleus and softer, outer epinucleus in a process called hydrodelineation (see Procedure, Hydrodelineation). This process allows for removal of the hard endonucleus first, within the capsular bag, using the epinucleus and cortex as a cushion to protect the underlying posterior capsule. The hard endonucleus is divided into several small pieces (the phaco fracture technique is described in the following section), which allows for a more controlled removal using less phacoemulsification power and less phacoemulsification time. These techniques require a continuous curvilinear capsulorrhexis to provide an intact and very resilient capsular opening. Because the nucleus is divided into pieces before removal from the capsular bag, the capsular opening can be smaller than with whole-nucleus removal. Effective hydrodissection and hydrodelineation are critical to the success of these techniques.

We are indebted to the many skillful and innovative surgeons who have developed these techniques, and we regret that we are unable to highlight and credit each and every technical variation. A working knowledge of many techniques is extremely helpful to the phacoemulsification surgeon, who can respond to unplanned situations that may arise during surgery by changing technique or approach.

Phaco fracture technique Building on the work of Gimbel, John Shephard developed a useful technique for hard nuclei: the 4-quadrant nucleofractis technique. After adequate hydrodissection and hydrodelineation, a deep central linear groove or trough is sculpted in the nucleus. Starting centrally, a linear groove is made in the axis of the incision. The nucleus is then rotated clockwise 90° within the bag (usually with the second instrument inserted through the paracentesis), and another linear groove is created perpendicular to the first. The nucleus is rotated clockwise, and the process repeated until four grooves are created. Each groove must be deep enough to allow subsequent cracking. Clues that the groove depth is adequate include smoothing of the striations in the groove, brightening of the red reflex in the groove, and sculpting to a depth of 2–3 phaco tip diameters.

Nuclear cracking can be done as each quadrant is created or after all 4 grooves have been placed. Cracking after all 4 grooves have been created seems to facilitate nuclear rotation. The phaco tip and second instrument are inserted into each groove and spread apart, with either a cross action or parallel action, thereby cracking the nucleus into 4 quarters.

The second instrument can then be used to elevate the apex of the quadrant while pushing the blunt periphery down (Figs 8-27A,B). The phaco tip engages the elevated apex, and, after adequate vacuum is attained, the nuclear quadrant is pulled toward the center of the capsular bag and emulsified. Each quadrant is sequentially removed in the same manner. Alternatively, the second instrument pushes the apex of the quadrant posteriorly so the peripheral rim moves anteriorly and toward the center, where it is engaged by the phaco tip and emulsified (Fig 8-27C). If the capsulotomy is small and a given nuclear quadrant is greater than 90°, care should be taken not to tear the capsule as the nuclear material is brought out of the bag. This is particularly true if the nucleus is hard. Alternatively, the fragment can be thinned out while still in the capsular bag.

Chopping techniques

The *phaco chop technique* originally described by Nagahara did not entail the creation of a central groove. He advocated using the natural fault lines in the lens nucleus to create a fracture plane. After burying the phaco tip in the center of the nucleus, the surgeon inserts a phaco chop instrument under the anterior capsular flap, impales the midperipheral nucleus inferiorly, and draws it toward the phaco tip, thereby cracking the nucleus into two pieces. This is termed *horizontal chopping*. The phaco tip is then buried in one of the nuclear halves, and the phaco chop instrument is used in traditional fashion to create multiple small wedges of nucleus for emulsification.

Koch and Katzen modified this procedure with the addition of a central groove because they encountered difficulty in mobilizing the nuclear fragments. The groove

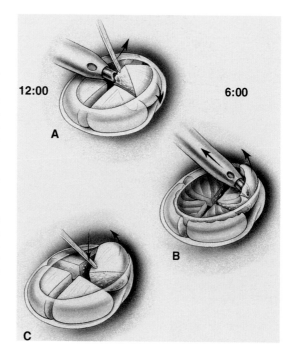

Figure 8-27 Quadrant management. **A**, Spatula lifts the apex of the quadrant, the ultrasound tip is embedded into the posterior edge, and aspiration centralizes the quadrant for emulsification. **B**, Quadrants are debulked centrally after splitting; the ultrasound tip is embedded into the cortical rim and aspiration is maintained to tumble the rim and remainder of the quadrant centrally. **C**, Spatula pushes the apex of the quadrant posteriorly so the rim moves to front and center. *(Reproduced with permission from Johnson SH. Phacoemulsification. Focal Points: Clinical Modules for Ophthalmologists. San Francisco: American Academy of Ophthalmology; 1994, module 6. Illustration by Christine Gralapp.)*

affords the surgeon more room to manipulate the nuclear pieces in the capsular bag. More recently, Nagahara's original technique has gained popularity because of both the use of more advanced phacoemulsification machines and the emergence of supracapsular phaco techniques that remove the whole nucleus from the confines of the capsular bag (see later in this section).

The chopping technique as popularized by Koch is a variation of divide and conquer (Fig 8-28). After adequate hydrodissection, deep nuclear sculpting is performed in the axis of the incision, creating a trough. A second instrument, designed for phaco chop, is inserted through the paracentesis, and the nucleus is cracked in half using either cross action or parallel action. The trough is rotated horizontally. If the surgeon is right-

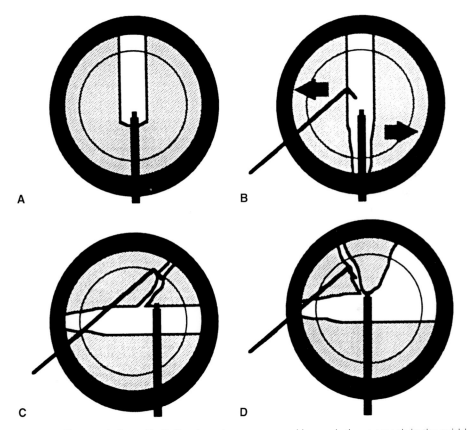

A

B

C

D

Figure 8-28 Stop and chop. **A**, Soft cataracts are prepared by sculpting a trench in the middle of the cataract, providing space for later manipulation. **B**, After sculpting is complete, the nucleus is fractured into two halves with the phaco tip and the chopper. **C**, The phaco tip is driven into the nuclear half about a third of the way across from right to left. The chopper is buried in the periphery of the nucleus and pulled toward the phaco tip. When the instruments are close to each other, they are separated, and a small segment of the nucleus is chopped off. It is already impaled on the phaco tip and can be emulsified without further manipulation. **D**, The phaco tip is driven into the remaining nucleus and the same steps are repeated: bury the chopper, pull it toward the phaco tip, chop, separate, remove. This sequence is repeated until the entire nucleus is emulsified. *(Reproduced with permission from Koch PS, Katzen LE. Stop and chop phacoemulsification. J Cataract Refract Surg. 1994;20:566–570. ©American Society of Cataract and Refractive Surgery.)*

handed, the phaco tip is then embedded to the right of center of the inferior nuclear half for stabilization (a left-handed surgeon would engage the nuclear half to the left). The phaco chop instrument is inserted underneath the anterior capsular edge in the lower right quadrant, advanced out to the periphery of the epinucleus, embedded in the peripheral epinucleus, and pulled back to the phaco tip, creating a small, free wedge of nucleus, which is easily emulsified and aspirated. The same piece of nucleus is again stabilized with the phaco tip, while the phaco chop instrument is advanced out to the periphery and pulled centrally, creating another small, free wedge of nucleus for emulsification and aspiration. The process is repeated until the entire first nuclear half is removed. The other nuclear half is rotated into the inferior capsular bag, and the process is repeated.

The size of the nuclear wedges can vary, depending on nuclear consistency; hard nuclei require smaller wedges, whereas softer nuclei can be safely removed with larger wedges. The advantages of this technique over conventional divide and conquer include reduced stress on the capsular bag and zonular fibers, decreased phacoemulsification power and time, and greater ease in dealing with very hard nuclei. High levels of vacuum are necessary to maintain a firm grasp on the nucleus as it is being fragmented; in addition, the high vacuum allows more controlled removal of the pieces and reduces the use of ultrasound energy. Any remaining epinucleus and cortex are removed in standard fashion.

More recently, some surgeons have begun to favor using the chopper centrally, within the pupillary space, to perform the initial crack. After impaling the nucleus with the phaco tip, the chopper is buried just adjacent to the phaco tip at the visual axis and drawn back toward the side port until the nucleus separates into halves. This procedure eliminates the sometimes dangerous placement of the chopper under the capsulorrhexis or the necessity of creating a groove. It has been termed *vertical chop* or *quick chop* and should be attempted with a chopper specifically designed for this technique.

The *supracapsular phaco technique,* described in 1997 by W.F. Maloney, also requires a large capsulorrhexis. This technique uses hydrodissection to elevate the nucleus completely out of the capsular bag. Some proponents recommend using a cohesive viscoelastic for hydrodissection to allow for better cleaving of the cortical–capsular attachments. After one pole of the nucleus is elevated, the hydrodissection tip is used to flip the nucleus over so the posterior surface of the nucleus faces anteriorly. The nucleus is then placed back into the posterior chamber but *above* the anterior capsular rim. The surgeon then continues on to perform his or her preferred nuclear splitting and removal procedures. The purported benefits of this technique are the reduced stress on the zonules, the relative ease and safety of cracking the nucleus because the phaco chop instrument does not need to be passed under the capsulorrhexis rim, and the ability to use this technique in patients with small pupils. The risks of this technique include a greater chance of aspirating and damaging the iris in the phaco tip (because the anterior capsular rim no longer separates the nucleus from the iris) and the greater need to maintain control of the nuclear pieces as they are created, because they are no longer contained in the capsular bag.

Nuclear flip techniques

Recently, Brown has described a variation on earlier supracapsular techniques. After creating a large, continuous curvilinear capsulorrhexis, the surgeon performs hydrodissection in the standard fashion with a blunt-tipped cannula. During this process, the lens is flipped into the anterior chamber, where it is emulsified.

Fine IH. The chip and flip phacoemulsification technique. *J Cataract Refract Surg.* 1991; 17:366–371.

Fine IH, Maloney WF, Dillman DM. Crack and flip phacoemulsification technique. *J Cataract Refract Surg.* 1993;19:797–802.

Gimbel HV. Divide and conquer nucleofractis phacoemulsification: development and variations. *J Cataract Refract Surg.* 1991;17:281–291.

Koch PS. *Mastering Phacoemulsification: A Simplified Manual of Strategies for the Spring, Crack, and Stop and Chop Technique.* 4th ed. Thorofare, NJ: Slack; 1994.

Koch PS. *Converting to Phacoemulsification: Making the Transition to In-the-Bag Phaco.* 3rd ed. Thorofare, NJ: Slack; 1992.

Koch PS, Davison JA, eds. *Textbook of Advanced Phacoemulsification Techniques.* Thorofare, NJ: Slack; 1991.

Shepherd JR. In situ fracture. *J Cataract Refract Surg.* 1990;16:436–440.

Steinert RF, ed. *Cataract Surgery: Techniques, Complications, and Management.* 2nd ed. St. Louis: Mosby; 2004.

Instrument settings for phacoemulsification

As described in previous sections, most methods of nucleus removal consist of several distinct steps, including sculpting, cracking, grasping, and emulsifying.

With contemporary phacoemulsification machines, all of the phacoemulsification parameters—power, aspiration flow rate, and vacuum—can be adjusted for each step of the procedure, giving the surgeon maximum control of the process. Table 8-1 shows suggested instrument settings for the basic steps in phacoemulsification. Because optimal instrument settings depend on the individual surgeon's technique and equipment, this table is presented for general reference only. *Sculpting,* the process of debulking the central nucleus, involves a shaving maneuver in which the tip of the phaco port is never fully occluded (Fig 8-29). Without occlusion, only incidental vacuum is generated. Only a

Table 8-1 Suggested Instrument Settings for Basic Steps Performed in Phacoemulsification

Hardness of Cataract	Vacuum Setting (Maximum)	Aspiration Flow Rate	Maximum Power
Sculpting nucleus before nuclear fracturing			
All types of cataract	40–60 mm Hg	20 cc/min	50%
Grasping/emulsifying divided nuclear fragments			
1+	70 mm Hg	25 cc/min	70%
2+	110 mm Hg	25 cc/min	70%
3+	150 mm Hg	25 cc/min	70%
4+	200 mm Hg	25 cc/min	70%

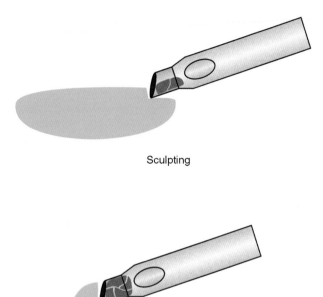

Figure 8-29 Sculpting versus occlusion. *(Reprinted with permission from Seibel BS.* Phacodynamics: Mastering the Tools and Techniques of Phacoemulsification Surgery. *3rd ed. Thorofare, NJ: Slack; 1999.)*

Sculpting

Occlusion

portion of the phaco needle is in contact with the nucleus with each forward pass; thus, lens material can be removed in a controlled fashion. *Aspiration,* the suctioning of fluid, is responsible for bringing the nuclear particles into the aspiration port and out of the eye. Sculpting is usually performed with minimal vacuum, low aspiration flow, and low phacoemulsification power.

Low vacuum is indicated for sculpting. Vacuum can be undesirable when the surgeon is sculpting near the periphery of the nucleus because large amounts of epinucleus or iris tissue can be pulled into the tip. Using low vacuum also allows for safer sculpting close to the posterior capsule both in eyes with small pupils and in patients with pseudoexfoliation, where zonular integrity may be abnormal. For all types of cataracts, sculpting usually requires low vacuum settings.

After the nucleus has been sculpted and cracked, the nuclear fragments are grasped and emulsified by occlusion of the phaco tip. Vacuum is essential at this point in the procedure to grasp the nuclear fragments, pull them to the center of the lens capsule, and emulsify them. Full occlusion of the phaco tip allows the vacuum to build up to its maximum preset level. Full vacuum draws nuclear material up into the tip and allows it to be deformed as it enters. The ultrasound power then emulsifies the material into smaller pieces. Flow functions to drive the emulsified nuclear material farther into the tip, and it also helps to feed additional nuclear material into the tip. The repulsive action of the ultrasound tip oscillating against the nuclear material is counterbalanced by the vacuum and the flow pulling the material inward.

The vacuum is set to a level appropriate for the hardness of the nucleus: harder cataracts require higher vacuum. If vacuum is set too low, lens chatter can occur, with large and small nuclear fragments bouncing around the anterior chamber. Higher vacuum improves the purchase of the phaco tip on the nuclear material and reduces ultrasound power and ultrasound time.

A low flow rate is considered desirable because it provides greater stability to the anterior chamber. After each nuclear fragment is completely emulsified and aspirated, and occlusion is broken, low flow is immediately resumed. With low flow, emulsification and aspiration occur at a slower, more controlled rate; with high flow, events occur more quickly, and iris and other intraocular tissue can be aspirated inadvertently.

This discussion is only a guideline to the basic parameters of phacoemulsification. Each surgeon must determine the best settings to use based on the particular machine and the surgical technique to be used for any given patient.

Irrigation and aspiration

The instruments and techniques for irrigation and aspiration in phacoemulsification are the same as for ECCE with manual expression. Occasionally, a small rim of nuclear or epinuclear material remains after phacoemulsification, and the surgeon may remove this soft material by crushing it into the aspiration port with a second instrument, while applying maximum vacuum suction. Alternatively, this epinuclear material may be removed with the phaco tip, using aspiration and occasional bursts of phacoemulsification power as needed.

The remaining anterior capsule may cause difficulty during removal of the peripheral cortical material of the lens. The surgeon can resolve this problem by rotating the port toward the equator of the lens capsule. The cortical material should be engaged under low suction and dragged to the center of the inflated capsular bag. The port is then rotated so that it is fully visible to the surgeon, and the remaining cortical material can be stripped under maximum suction.

Sometimes the surgeon finds it difficult to reach the subincisional cortex closest to and underlying the wound. In these cases, a 45°, right-angle (90°), or U-shaped (180°) aspiration cannula may be useful to engage and strip this problematic cortical material. The aspiration cannula can be attached either to a handheld syringe or to the irrigation/aspiration handpiece. Some surgeons still prefer the simplicity and control of a manual system for routine cortical cleanup, either with a single- or double-bore cannula or a bimanual system.

If some residual cortex is resistant to removal, the intraocular lens can be inserted to open the capsular bag and keep the posterior capsule away from the aspiration port. Some surgeons also rotate the IOL so the haptics will further loosen the cortex. (Intraocular lenses are discussed in detail beginning with the section Primary Intraocular Lens Implantation in Adults.) The benefits of attempting to remove small amounts of residual cortex must be weighed against the risk of damaging the posterior capsule. Small amounts of residual cortex may be easily resorbed.

Types of Cataract Surgery: Laser Phacolysis

Although ultrasonic phacoemulsification is a safe means of removing a cataract in most cases, some surgeons feel the process can be made even safer. To this end, physicians and device makers have developed laser phacolysis. Laser phacolysis systems use either Nd:YAG or Er:YAG laser handpieces to break up nuclear material, either by direct ablation (Photon Laser Phacoemulsification System, Paradigm Medical Industries, Salt Lake City) or by way of acoustic shock waves created when the laser strikes a metal stop at the end of the handpiece (Dodick Photolysis System, A.R.C. Laser Corp, Salt Lake City).

At present, the systems offer two primary advantages: (1) They produce no clinically significant heat at the site of the entry incision, which decreases the risk of corneal or scleral burns. (2) Because no heat is produced, the handpieces don't require thick cooling sleeves or irrigation lines to protect against burns. This allows them to operate through small incisions, less than 2 mm in width. A possible third advantage is that the systems are safer for intraocular structures such as the endothelium and posterior capsule because they release less energy from the tip; more research is required before this can be verified.

The disadvantage of the systems as currently configured appears to be their difficulty in easily emulsifying harder cataracts. They may not be as effective as ultrasonic phaco-emulsification when faced with a cataract of grade 3+ and higher. As a backup, most laser phacolysis systems are also equipped with an ultrasonic probe so the surgeon can convert to conventional phacoemulsification.

Clear Lens Extraction

Recently, some surgeons have advocated clear lens extraction, with implantation of high-power IOLs in patients with high hyperopia, and very low or even minus-power IOLs in patients with high myopia. For a discussion of techniques, risks, and benefits of this procedure, see Chapter 10, Cataract Surgery in Special Situations.

Pars Plana Lensectomy

The posterior approach to lens extraction is performed through the pars plana, generally in combination with vitrectomy.

Indications

The presence of a significant cataract with the urgent need for pars plana vitrectomy and/or retinal surgery is the general indication for this approach. Following trauma with lens rupture and vitreous disruption, this single approach is the best way to clean all of the vitreous and lens material from the eye. A pars plana approach may also facilitate removal of retained foreign bodies and management of perforating injuries. Crystalline lens removal may be essential in procedures for anterior proliferation of the hyaloid and in cases requiring anterior dissection of the vitreous for detachments with proliferative vitreoretinopathy. A posterior approach may be desirable in cases of symptomatic lens subluxation.

Contraindications

The most common contraindication for this approach is a nucleus too hard to be removed by this technique. Most cataracts with brunescent nuclear sclerosis are unsuitable for fragmentation through the pars plana even though it may be possible to safely perform phacoemulsification by the anterior approach. In such cases, a procedure combining anterior cataract extraction and pars plana vitrectomy may be considered when surgery is urgent. If delay of the posterior segment procedure is appropriate, sequential procedures can minimize the anterior segment inflammatory reaction present at the time of the retinal and vitreous surgery.

Instrumentation

Standard vitrectomy instrumentation is adequate for removing the lens capsule and cortex in children and young adults. With a firm nucleus, ultrasonic fragmentation is required. The instrument used for pars plana lens fragmentation is narrower than that used for anterior segment extraction and does not require coaxial infusion because vitrectomy is generally performed with a separate infusion line.

Procedure

After the standard pars plana ports are established, the posterior lens capsule is opened. The lens fragmentation needle is introduced through the capsule opening, and the nucleus is emulsified in multiple strokes. The suction cutter is used to remove lens cortex, capsule, and debris. Small pieces of nucleus that are too hard to be aspirated or cut can be broken into smaller fragments and aspirated by using a second instrument to push the pieces against the cutter port.

Primary Intraocular Lens Implantation in Adults

Historical Perspective

In the late 1940s, the first modern intraocular lens—the disk-shaped Ridley lens—was developed. Since that time, lens design has undergone many modifications, as researchers have developed, used, and discarded lens designs in a continuing evolution toward a better lens (Figure 8-30).

The history of IOL implantation, however, begins long before the 1940s. The first reported IOL implant occurred in 1795, when Casaamata, an ophthalmologist in Dresden, attempted to use an IOL to correct aphakic vision. The results were not successful, and no further attempts were reported until 150 years later.

Kirby DB. *Surgery of Cataract.* Philadelphia: Lippincott; 1950:11.

The development of modern IOL implantation began in 1949. Harold Ridley, an English ophthalmologist, observed that polymethylmethacrylate (PMMA) fragments

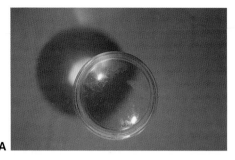

A

Original Ridley lens, first implanted by Harold Ridley in November 1949.

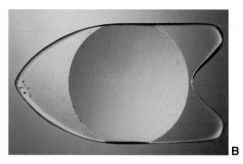

B

Angle-supported lens designed by Strampelli; used from 1950 to 1955.

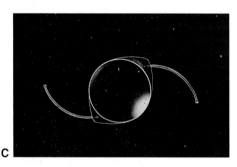

C

Anterior chamber lens designed by Joaquin Barraquer; haptics made of nylon were implanted in anterior chamber angle.

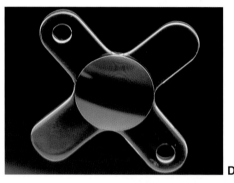

D

Epstein lens made by Copeland; iris-supported with 2 opposing haptics placed anterior and posterior to the iris.

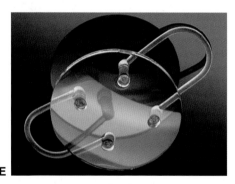

E

Two-loop iris-fixated lens designed by Binkhorst; lens was inserted after extracapsular surgery, with haptics posterior to the iris in the capsular bag; fibrosis then fixated lens in place.

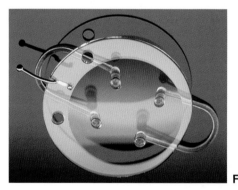

F

Medallion lens with platinum clip designed by Worst; lens was implanted with polypropylene haptics posterior to the iris at 6 and 12 o'clock; peripheral iridectomy was made, and the platinum clip was bent back against the superior haptic to secure the lens against dislocation.

Figure 8-30 Historical intraocular lenses. *(Photographs courtesy of Robert C. Drews, MD.)*

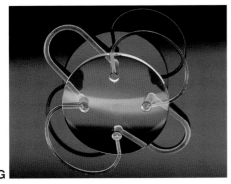

G

Original iris-fixated lens designed by Fyodorov, as made in the United States; 2 looped haptics were placed posterior to the iris, and the optic and 2 opposing loops were placed anterior to the iris.

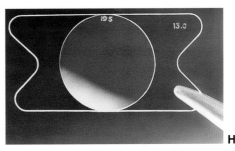

H

Mark VIII lens designed by Choyce; rigid lens was implanted in anterior chamber angle either as a secondary lens implant or primarily after intracapsular cataract surgery.

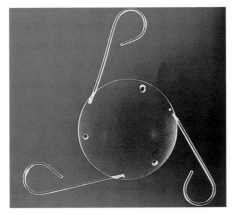

I

Anterior chamber lens designed by Copeland; haptics were made of polypropylene and were flexible enough to conform to chamber angle independently of corneal diameter.

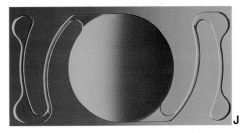

J

Kelman open-looped anterior chamber lens; optic vaulted anteriorly, and haptics were planar and situated in the anterior chamber angle.

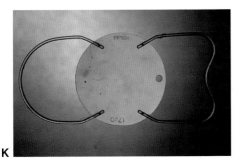

K

Azar 91Z lens; designed to be placed with rounded haptic in inferior chamber angle and notched haptic in superior chamber angle, with lens vaulted anteriorly.

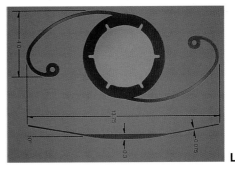

L

Lens made by Lynell; featured a glass optic and could be autoclaved.

Figure 8-30 *(Continued)*

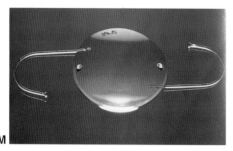

M

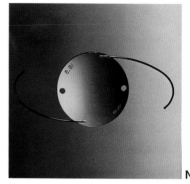

N

J-loop posterior chamber lens designed by Shearing; designed to be used with either extracapsular cataract surgery or phacoemulsification and to be placed in capsular bag or ciliary sulcus.

Modified J-loop lens designed by Sinskey; early models had 2 positioning holes to facilitate placement in capsular bag; haptics were made of polypropylene initially, and optic was made of PMMA.

Plate haptic silicone IOL designed by Mazzocco; designed to fit into capsular bag or ciliary sulcus; lens migration occurred in some cases after posterior capsulotomy.

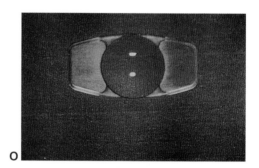

O

Figure 8-30 *(Continued)*

from airplane cockpit windshields were well tolerated in the anterior segment of the eyes of pilots. He placed a disk-shaped PMMA lens into the posterior chamber of a 45-year-old woman after performing an ECCE.

Ridley's lens corrected aphakic vision, but a high incidence of postoperative complications such as glaucoma, uveitis, and dislocation caused him to abandon his lens design. Though frustrated in his attempts, Ridley showed foresight in three important areas. First, he constructed his original lens of PMMA in a biconvex design. Second, he used extracapsular surgery for implantation of the lens. Third, he placed the lens in the posterior chamber behind the iris.

Ophthalmologists in the 1950s were troubled by the serious complications associated with early IOL styles and by the fact that nearly all of the investigative work was done in humans, occasionally with very little scientific basis. Uncertainty concerning the long-term success and stability of these lenses limited their use. Yet the desire to manage aphakia without the problems and inconvenience of aphakic spectacles or contact lenses continued to inspire investigation into IOL implantation. After the failure of the Ridley lens, most surgeons turned their interests to anterior chamber lenses.

Extracapsular cataract surgery in the 1950s was crude by modern standards and was generally associated with retained lens cortex, which caused fibrosis and adhesions between iris and capsule. Intracapsular cataract extraction (ICCE) eliminated residual cortical material and became the preferred procedure. Thus, structures for fixation of the IOLs of the 1950s used haptics that extended beyond the optical portion of the lens into the anterior chamber angle for support.

Anterior chamber lenses were of 2 principal types: those with flexible supports made of nylon and those with rigid supports made of PMMA. These lenses failed in the first instance because of disintegration of the haptics and in the second because of inflammation and compromised angle structures. The prototype of flexible supports was the Dannheim lens (1955), and the prototype of rigid supports was the Strampelli lens (1953). Epstein of South Africa turned to the Maltese cross design, which was intended to have 2 haptics behind the iris and 2 haptics in front. This lens was later modified by Copeland. The early Copeland lens resulted in a 15% incidence of cystoid macular edema because of iris movement over the haptics of the lens, with pupillary constriction and dilation.

Binkhorst of the Netherlands first designed a lens in 1957 to clip onto the iris and minimize iris chafe. In 1969, Worst, a pupil of Binkhorst, began to suture the Binkhorst lens to the iris in an effort to decrease dislocation. The Worst lens was a modification of the Binkhorst lens that used a platinum clip bent through the iridectomy as a means of attaching the lens to the iris. Many styles of iris clip lenses were developed and inserted before surgeons began to notice a high incidence of uveitis, glaucoma, and hyphema (UGH syndrome). This syndrome was evident with several early types of anterior chamber lenses as well. Some iris clip lenses had a tendency to dislocate into the vitreous upon pupillary dilation. Corneal decompensation secondary to corneal touch was another important complication. Iris clip lenses were completely abandoned until their more recent reincarnation for refractive surgery.

In England in the early 1960s, Choyce made a number of modifications to the original Strampelli lens. The result was a series of IOLs that were known as the Choyce Mark I through Mark VIII lenses. The Choyce Mark VIII lens was subsequently modified and manufactured as the Tennant lens.

Azar designed a modification of the Choyce lens, substituting a single footplate inferiorly and a double footplate superiorly that became known as the Azar lens. A flexible modification of this rigid lens, manufactured as the Kelman lens, had 3-point fixation with a measure of flexibility with the inferior arm.

Joaquin Barraquer modified the Dannheim lens to get more flexibility in the anterior chamber angle. Years later, in the 1980s, Shearing reintroduced Barraquer's modification of the Dannheim lens with polypropylene loops for use in the posterior chamber following ECCE.

Design Considerations

Rigid anterior chamber lenses could be used with either ICCE or ECCE, but fitting the length of the lens to the width of the chamber was difficult. The IOL length was selected by estimating anterior chamber width based on the horizontal corneal diameter. Because such estimation is crude even with modern instruments, complications arose. Overly long IOLs were painful, and short lenses would decenter or rotate. At first, intractable uveitis resulted from manufacturing techniques, but even improved manufacturing techniques failed to eliminate secondary glaucoma, cystoid macular edema, and bullous keratopathy resulting from poorly fitted IOLs.

Complications associated with rigid anterior chamber IOLs spurred the development of the flexible-loop anterior chamber IOL. This device evolved into a lens optic positioned in front of the pupil by flexible extensions or polypropylene loops, which would sit in the angle.

In the 1980s, attempts to make more flexible loops in the anterior chamber that would not dissolve led to the popular Leiske lens and the Azar 91Z lens, which were flexible manifestations of Strampelli's design that used manufacturing materials and methods current in the 1980s. Designs with closed loops were subsequently found to produce forward movement of the optic and flexing of the loops with corneal contact, resulting in significantly increased late complications. Most of these IOL designs were withdrawn or abandoned, and today closed-loop anterior chamber IOLs are generally removed from eyes at the earliest sign of trouble. The more successful anterior chamber lens designs involve open loops or S- and Z-shaped loops with 3 or 4 points of contact within the angle.

As ECCE, and later phacoemulsification, became the standard for cataract surgery in the 1980s, anterior chamber IOLs were largely relegated to a backup role, used when capsular rupture or other problems precluded implantation of a posterior chamber IOL.

Explantation studies of anterior chamber lenses since the mid-1950s have shown that most anterior chamber lenses produced results inferior to those of posterior chamber lenses. Higher incidences of retinal detachment and cystoid macular edema shaped the clinical perception that emerged in the 1980s that anterior chamber lenses were inferior to posterior chamber lenses. Many complications attributed to anterior chamber lenses during this period, however, were actually caused by the complications of unplanned extracapsular surgery. Today, modern flexible anterior chamber lenses are felt by most surgeons to be a safe and acceptable alternative to sutured posterior chamber lenses (see Posterior Chamber IOLs).

Apple DJ, Mamalis N, Olson RJ, et al. *Intraocular Lenses: Evolution, Designs, Complications, and Pathology.* Baltimore: Williams & Wilkins; 1989.

Posterior Chamber IOLs

Expanded awareness of the role the endothelium plays in corneal clarity was a factor in the evolution of posterior chamber IOL implantation. The dramatic rise in the incidence of pseudophakic bullous keratopathy was documented in numerous papers reporting the shifting indication for keratoplasty at major corneal centers. The discovery that viscous sodium hyaluronate could protect the endothelium from critical damage during IOL implantation was a turning point in the acceptance of IOLs by the ophthalmic community. Sodium hyaluronate and other viscoelastic substances facilitate lens insertion, reduce operative complications, and hasten visual recovery by minimizing striate keratopathy in the early postoperative period. These substances stabilize the anterior chamber depth during capsulotomy for the ECCE surgeon and ease the transition into ECCE and phacoemulsification. The use of viscoelastic remains the standard for routine cataract surgery in the United States. (For more detailed discussion, see Viscoelastics later in this chapter.)

With the advent of microsurgical techniques and the operating microscope, extracapsular surgery became much more precise. Initially, both rigid and flexible lenses were placed in the anterior chamber following extracapsular surgery, although the placement of a lens in the posterior chamber became more feasible. Shearing modified the flexible version of the second Strampelli lens for posterior chamber placement. Subsequent modifications of this lens by Pierce, Sinskey, and Shearing elevated ECCE with posterior chamber lens implantation to the position of standard procedure.

Posterior chamber IOLs evolved concurrently with advances in instrumentation and technique for ECCE and phacoemulsification. Originally designed with a disk-shaped optic stabilized by polypropylene J-loops, these IOLs have undergone numerous geometric changes: loops have varied in length, stiffness, vault, and angle configuration; and optics have varied in diameter, shape, positioning holes, and manufacturing style.

The positioning of the IOL in the eye also influenced lens design. Because can-opener capsulotomy did not always result in a stable capsular bag to hold both loops of the implant, surgeons sometimes experienced difficulty positioning the loops symmetrically, either in the capsule or in the ciliary sulcus. Some manufacturers attempted to resolve the problem by designing IOLs with asymmetric loops for placement of the inferior loop in the capsule and the superior loop in the ciliary sulcus. The technique of rotating, or "dialing," the IOL into position created a need for "left-handed" lenses that could be rotated counterclockwise by left-handed surgeons. The problems of positioning the trailing loop plagued some surgeons learning posterior chamber lens insertion, leading to the development of eyelets and notches on 1 loop to allow placement using lens hooks. IOL decentration resulted in distortion of the visual image by the edge of the optic or the positioning holes. Many of these highly specific features have been abandoned as the surgical skills of cataract surgeons have become more refined.

IOL optic geometry has also evolved from the earlier planoconvex models to the newer biconvex design. Numerous changes in the shape of the posterior IOL surface were advanced to reduce late opacification of the crystalline lens capsule and to facilitate laser capsulotomy. "Laser ridges" rimming the posterior optic facilitate Nd:YAG laser capsulotomy by separating the capsule from the lens surface. Other lens modifications include the incorporation of ultraviolet-absorbing chromophores into the material of the IOL to protect the retina from actinic radiation. Special purpose lenses, such as those designed specifically for suture fixation in the ciliary sulcus, were also developed. These lenses have eyelets molded into the inside curve of the haptics to facilitate suture attachment. Other types of special-use IOLs include lenses designed with opaque flanges to decrease glare in clinical conditions such as aniridia and coloboma.

Oval optic designs were developed to allow insertion through the smaller incisions made possible by phacoemulsification. Because phacoemulsification wounds are generally less than 4 mm, and a solid optic with this diameter would not provide an adequate optical zone, a variety of foldable soft IOLs have been developed from a variety of materials. Those now available can be placed through incisions that measure 2.5–4.5 mm.

Mazzocco is generally given credit for developing a foldable intraocular lens. The obvious advantage of the foldable lens design is that it allows implantation of the IOL through a small incision. The availability of a small-incision lens coupled with the resurgence of phacoemulsification as a method of cataract extraction has resulted in the rapid and widespread popularity of these lenses. Although various materials have been evaluated, the majority of foldable lenses currently manufactured are fabricated from either silicone or acrylic materials.

Several designs of foldable IOLs are available, including the original Mazzocco "plate" style or the traditional flexible loop/haptic style derived from the original Shearing design. The flexible haptic designs may offer the advantage of increased stability in the capsular bag following laser posterior capsulotomy.

Although either silicone or acrylic materials are suitable for most patients, problems have been reported with silicone IOLs in patients undergoing vitrectomy with either air–fluid exchange or silicone oil injection. When cataract surgery is to be performed in a patient who is likely to require vitreoretinal surgery in the future, an IOL material other than silicone is preferred. In addition, early evidence suggests that the squared-edge optic design found initially in acrylic IOLs is associated with a lower rate of posterior capsular opacification and thus a reduced need for Nd:YAG capsulotomy.

Hollick EJ, Spalton DJ, Ursell PG, et al. The effect of polymethylmethacrylate, silicone, and polyacrylic intraocular lenses on posterior capsular opacification 3 years after cataract surgery. *Ophthalmology.* 1999;106:49–54.

Multifocal Lenses

One of the major drawbacks of intraocular lenses as a replacement for the human crystalline lens has been the fixed focus of the IOL. Although patients may see well at distance following cataract surgery, reading spectacles are generally required for near work. To address this issue, multifocal IOLs that provide refractive correction for both near and distance vision are now available, with others under investigation. These lenses offer an optical compromise: increased depth of focus in exchange for loss of contrast acuity.

The original bifocal IOL concept was based on the principle that the pupil tends to constrict for near tasks, so the central portion of the lens was designed for near and the outer portion for distance. The obvious disadvantage is that distance correction is not available when bright lights constrict the pupil. More recent designs address this problem with central and outer zones for distance correction and intermediate zones for near. Other designs have aspheric portions or multiple annular zones to provide a continuous variation in refractive power. A combination of geometric optics and diffraction optics can also achieve a multifocal effect, and the long-term effects of multifocal lenses are under investigation.

The drawbacks of multifocal IOLs include loss of contrast sensitivity, loss of best-corrected visual acuity, glare and halos, and more "chair time" spent counseling these patients. The advantages include bilateral stereoscopic vision and improved visual function at all distances without glasses. Multifocal IOLs require very accurate biometry and IOL calculations, and they work best in patients with minimal astigmatism. CNS adaptation to multifocal IOLs is best when the second eye is done 1–2 weeks after the first.

Although clinical experience with these lenses is still somewhat limited, data are available indicating that patients who have received bilateral multifocal lens implants report an improved quality of life. Patient selection is very important to ensure success with multifocal lenses, as the loss of contrast acuity and sharp distance focus can be very disconcerting for some patients, such as those with macular disease. (See also BCSC Section 3, *Clinical Optics.*) Some surgeons have reported a higher than usual explantation rate with these lenses.

Javitt JC, Wang F, Trentacost DJ, et al. Outcomes of cataract extraction with multifocal intraocular lens implantation: functional status and quality of life. *Ophthalmology.* 1997;104:589–599.

Nichamin LD. IOL update: new materials, designs, selection criteria, and insertion techniques. *Focal Points: Clinical Modules for Ophthalmologists.* San Francisco: American Academy of Ophthalmology; 1999, module 11.

Other Designs

Several new FDA-approved IOLs have been introduced with special attributes that may benefit patients if additional clinical experience proves them effective. Toric IOLs have been available from STAAR Surgical for a few years on a silicone plate haptic platform. The tendency of the lens to rotate in situ and its limited power options have kept this lens from being more widely adopted. Although lenses with ultraviolet chromophores have been standard for several decades, a blue blocker has been added to Alcon's latest entry in the silicone market. The Tecnis lens by Pharmacia provides a wavefront-designed optic that mimics the prolate shape of the natural lens and is touted to improve contrast sensitivity.

Phakic IOLs

The use of IOLs is not limited solely to the correction of aphakia. With increased interest in refractive surgery and appreciation of the significant disabilities caused by high refractive errors (both myopic and hyperopic), IOLs have been recognized as therapeutic options for the correction of refractive errors without concomitant cataract. The treatment of high myopia (over −12 D to −14 D) and high hyperopia (over +5 D to +6 D) with laser technology has been less than optimal due to loss of image quality and optical aberrations; a major advantage of implanted lenses is their ability to satisfactorily correct such high refractive errors. Another significant advantage of IOLs for the correction of refractive errors is their adjustability and reversibility. In the event that the patient is either over- or undercorrected, the lens can be exchanged; and if the correction is unsatisfactory, the lens can be removed and the patient returned to the pre-IOL refractive state. The use of refractive IOLs is also attractive from a technical standpoint, in that most ophthalmologists in the United States today are more comfortable with the surgical techniques of IOLs than with some of the newer refractive technologies. However, because the placement of a phakic IOL is an intraocular procedure, the risks inherent in all intraocular surgery, such as endophthalmitis, hemorrhage, and retinal detachment, must be considered.

IOLs have been designed for implantation in the phakic patient for the purpose of correcting both myopia and hyperopia. There are 3 general design types. The first is the posterior chamber lens. These are plate-type lenses made of hydrogel polymers that fit behind the iris in the ciliary sulcus. Ideally, these lenses should have some anterior vault so that crystalline lens–iris touch is avoided. Complications with this lens design include decentration, pupillary block glaucoma, and cataract formation. The second design is an anterior chamber iris clip lens. Unlike the iris clip IOLs used in cataract surgery in the 1970s and 1980s, which were clipped to the iris through the pupil, the phakic iris clip IOLs lie entirely within the anterior chamber and attach to the peripheral iris by means of 2 "claws." This design derives from a lens designed by Worst for aphakic correction. Complications with the iris claw lens include iritis, endothelial cell loss, and decentration. The third type is an adaptation of current pseudophakic anterior chamber lens styles. Problems encountered with this type of lens include ovalization of the pupil and iritis.

Patient experience with these lenses remains limited to date, and clinical trials to evaluate them are in progress in the United States. Although phakic IOLs appear promising as adjuncts to the refractive surgical armamentarium, their safety and effectiveness for long-term correction of refractive errors remain unknown.

Fechner PU, Haigis W, Wichmann W. Posterior chamber myopia lenses in phakic eyes. *J Cataract Refract Surg.* 1996;22:178–182.

Fechner PU, Haubitz I, Wichmann W, et al. Worst-Fechner biconcave minus power phakic iris-claw lens. *J Refract Surg.* 1999;15:93–105.

O'Brien TP, Awwad ST. Phakic intraocular lenses and refractive lensectomy for myopia. *Curr Opin Ophthalmol.* 2002;13:264–270.

Sanders DR, Martin RG, Brown DC, et al. Posterior chamber phakic intraocular lens for hyperopia. *J Refract Surg.* 1999;15:309–315.

IOL Power Determination

In the United States, IOLs are implanted in more than 98% of all cataract extractions. Of all the various methods of aphakic correction, IOL implantation provides the most natural visual function and convenience to the patient. The last decade has seen great improvements in the accuracy with which the surgeon can determine the IOL power required to achieve emmetropia. The development of better instrumentation for measuring the axial length (AL) of the eye and the use of more precise mathematical formulas to perform the appropriate calculations have contributed to these improvements. However, the surgeon must have a basic understanding of the relationship between the patient's previous refractive state and each of the measurement parameters in order to avoid errors in calculation.

The approximate IOL power needed to achieve emmetropia can be calculated quickly by starting with a power of 18 D and adding to it the patient's preoperative refractive state multiplied by 1.6 (use negative numbers for myopia and positive numbers for hyperopia). Patients who have induced myopia from nuclear sclerosis require more careful calculation, but if the surgeon has refraction records showing a stable reading, the reading can be used as a quick check on the calculated IOL power. This double check can avoid a large postoperative refractive error.

Regression formulas are used to predict the appropriate IOL power for emmetropia based on the refracting power of the cornea, the anticipated postoperative distance between the anterior surface of the cornea and the anterior surface of the IOL (anterior chamber depth), and the axial length of the eye. The refracting power of the cornea is determined with the keratometer. Anterior chamber depth is estimated from measurements made on eyes with implants similar to the style of IOL to be used. The axial length is the distance between the anterior surface of the cornea and the fovea as measured by A-scan ultrasonography.

The most widely used regression formula was developed by Sanders, Retzlaff, and Kraff and is known as the SRK formula:

$$P = A - (2.5L) - 0.9K$$

where

P = lens implant power for emmetropia (diopters)
L = axial length (mm)
K = average keratometric reading (diopters)
A = constant specific to the lens implant to be used

A constants for each IOL are specified by the manufacturer. The constant is a theoretical value that relates the lens power to axial length and keratometry. The A constant is generally between 113 for anterior chamber lenses and 119 for biconvex posterior chamber lenses. The A constant has no units and is specific to the design of the IOL and its intended location and orientation within the eye.

Regression formulas plot a linear relationship that approximates nonlinear data. Thus, for patients with high myopia and high hyperopia, the deviation of the expected value from the true value increases. The original regression formulas have now been modified to increase their accuracy based on clinical experience, and newer formulas account for these sources of error and also allow for calculation of powers for secondary IOLs and for IOLs not intended to produce emmetropia. Although previous regression formulas have depended on axial length and keratometry for the calculation, newer formulas (such as the Holladay II formula) incorporate measured anterior chamber depth, lens thickness, and corneal diameter to significantly increase the accuracy of the IOL calculation. These formulas and the related software are especially helpful in extremely short eyes, where piggyback IOLs are required to achieve emmetropia.

Fenzl RE, Gills JP, Cherchio M. Refractive and visual outcome of hyperopic cataract cases operated on before and after implementation of the Holladay II formula. *Ophthalmology.* 1998;105:1759–1764.

Hoffer KJ. Modern IOL power calculations: avoiding errors and planning for special circumstances. *Focal Points: Clinical Modules for Ophthalmologists.* San Francisco: American Academy of Ophthalmology; 1999, module 12.

Even though regression formulas can provide accurate predictions of IOL power for the majority of patients, several types of errors can be the source of significant postoperative refractive problems. Certainly, the measurements on which the calculation is based must be accurate. Errors in measuring corneal power can occur because of warpage from

recommended for IOL calculation, if possible, as this method may be the "safest"; that is, in case of a post-IOL refractive error, it is generally preferable to err on the myopic side. It is prudent, therefore, for the surgeon to discuss the difficult aspects of IOL calculations with any patients who have had refractive surgery.

As an example of the use of this method, consider a 45-year-old accountant who previously underwent LASIK. Good historical data are available and show the following numbers for the right eye: The preoperative average corneal power was measured by keratometry to be 44.75 D. The patient's spherical equivalent before refractive surgery was −6.50. His stable refractive error 1 year after surgery was −0.25. The net refractive change is −6.25 D, and thus his corrected corneal power after surgery is calculated to be 38.50 D. This number should be used as the average corneal power for IOL calculations.

Drews RC. Reliability of lens implant power formulas in hyperopes and myopes. *Ophthalmic Surg.* 1988;19:11–15.

Hoffer KJ. The Hoffer Q formula: a comparison of theoretic and regression formulas. *J Cataract Refract Surg.* 1993;19:700–712.

Holladay JT, Prager TC, Chandler TY, et al. A three-part system for refining intraocular lens power calculations. *J Cataract Refract Surg.* 1988;14:17–24.

Olsen T, Thim K, Corydon L. Theoretical versus SRK I and SRK II calculation of intraocular lens power. *J Cataract Refract Surg.* 1990;16:217–225.

Sanders DR, Retzlaff JA, Kraff MC. A-scan biometry and IOL implant power calculations. *Focal Points: Clinical Modules for Ophthalmologists.* San Francisco: American Academy of Ophthalmology; 1995, module 10.

Sanders DR, Retzlaff JA, Kraff MC, et al. Comparison of the SRK/T formula and other theoretical and regression formulas. *J Cataract Refract Surg.* 1990;16:341–346.

Seitz B, Langenbucher A, Nguyen NX, et al. Underestimation of intraocular lens power for cataract surgery after myopic photorefractive keratectomy. *Ophthalmology.* 1999;106:693–702.

Instrumentation

Polymethylmethacrylate (PMMA) IOLs may be safely handled with standard fine smooth forceps for insertion. Silicone and hydrogel IOLs must be handled more gently. Insertion forceps often have longer tips than do tying forceps to help in positioning across the anterior chamber.

Surgeons implanting a foldable lens use a variety of instruments to hold the IOL in its folded position during insertion and then to release it into the chamber. These instruments are of 2 general designs: (1) an injection tube that fits into the small wound and injects the IOL through the tube to unfold in the eye, and (2) molded forceps that hold the folded IOL as it slides through the small wound.

Lens glides are thin plastic sheets that can be placed in the eye to protect ocular structures from the IOL during insertion. They are typically used with anterior chamber lenses to avoid snagging the inferior pupil margin or iris as the IOL is positioned. When the leading haptic is in place, the lens glide is removed.

Once the IOL is implanted, its position can be adjusted with various lens hooks and manipulators if necessary. The most common is the Sinskey hook, a simple L-shaped hook used to adjust lens centration. Other hooks have front and back curves to manipulate the iris or lens capsule in relation to the IOL.

For patients with highly hyperopic eyes, a single IOL with sufficient power to produce emmetropia may not be available. In these cases, some surgeons have implanted 2 IOLs to generate sufficient convergent power. This technique is called *piggybacking* and can be performed with either PMMA or foldable lenses. In general, lenses are selected and placed so that the higher-power lens is more posterior in the capsular bag and the lower-power lens is either in the bag or in the sulcus. This positioning facilitates lens exchange of the lower-power IOL for refractive adjustment postoperatively if necessary. A potential complication of piggyback IOLs is the formation of interlenticular opacification, most commonly seen with acrylic IOLs, which has necessitated IOL explantation in some cases. It has not been reported with silicone IOLs to date or with silicone–acrylic combinations.

Gayton JL, Apple DJ, Peng Q, et al. Interlenticular opacification: clinicopathological correlation of a complication of posterior chamber piggyback intraocular lenses. *J Cataract Refract Surg.* 2000;26:330–336.

Gayton JL, Sanders VN. Implanting two posterior chamber intraocular lenses in a case of microphthalmos. *J Cataract Refract Surg.* 1993;19:776–777.

Procedure

The wound size must be large enough to accommodate the IOL. Larger wounds for intracapsular or extracapsular surgery are generally closed with sutures to obtain the appropriate opening size, whereas smaller wounds from phacoemulsification surgery may need to be enlarged if the IOL to be implanted is not folded. Viscoelastic or air is used to stabilize the anterior chamber depth and to protect the corneal endothelium from contact with the IOL. The microscope should be adjusted to give a full-field view of the eye. The globe is positioned so that the lens can be inserted with best visibility and access to the wound.

Posterior chamber IOL implantation

Posterior chamber IOLs may be secured within the capsular bag or in front of the capsule within the ciliary sulcus. Viscoelastic can be injected between the anterior and posterior capsule to expand this space. The IOL is advanced through the wound, with the leading haptic placed into position first (Fig 8-31A). The IOL optic is then brought into the pupil, and the trailing haptic is flexed and placed into position (Fig 8-31B). If a capsulorrhexis has been made, implantation can be performed with direct visualization of the anterior capsule opening. With other types of capsule opening, such as a can-opener capsulotomy, visualizing the anterior capsule for precise placement of the trailing haptic may be more difficult.

Foldable IOLs are inserted into the capsular bag with insertion forceps or an injector and then allowed to open in situ. For those foldable lenses with haptics, the superior loop is then flexed and placed into position within the capsular bag. Plate haptic design lenses are usually inserted into the capsular bag in toto with an injector; placing these lenses into the ciliary sulcus is unstable. The IOL position can be adjusted with a hook, and the lens may be rotated carefully to achieve adequate centration. Slight indentation of the sclera just posterior to the limbus should flex the loop without significantly altering centration. The viscoelastic is then aspirated to minimize the risk of postoperative intraocular pressure rise, and the anterior chamber depth is adjusted with balanced salt solution.

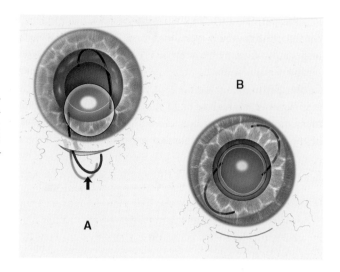

Figure 8-31 Posterior chamber IOL implantation. **A**, Inferior loop is placed in position. **B**, Superior loop is flexed and then placed in position. *(Illustration by Christine Gralapp.)*

Several techniques have been described for securing a posterior chamber IOL behind the iris with sutures when capsular support is inadequate. Transscleral polypropylene sutures may be used to secure the IOL haptics in the ciliary sulcus. Polypropylene sutures may also be used to attach posterior chamber IOL haptics or the optic to the overlying iris. Polypropylene sutures should be used instead of nylon sutures because nylon degrades over time, and lens dislocation may result. Suture fixation techniques are more difficult than standard implantation and are associated with a greater risk of complications (such as vitreous hemorrhage, dislocation, or late endophthalmitis). Sutured posterior chamber IOLs are most valuable as an alternative to anterior chamber IOL implantation in situations where an angle-supported lens might be considered problematic (for example, with keratoplasty, glaucoma-filtering surgery, or extensive peripheral anterior synechiae).

Anterior chamber IOL implantation

Anterior chamber IOLs are supported by the chamber angle and are generally flexible. Earlier rigid types of anterior chamber IOLs required precise sizing to avoid lens movement and erosion of adjacent tissues. Sizing of flexible lenses varies with the lens design. In the normal eye, the chamber angle is circular whereas the limbus is oval. It is common practice to use 1 mm plus the horizontal diameter of the limbus, as measured externally with a caliper ("white to white"), to determine the appropriate length for the anterior chamber IOL.

The pupil is generally constricted pharmacologically prior to IOL implantation. At least 1, and often 2, peripheral iridectomies are created to avoid pupillary block by the IOL optic. The anterior chamber depth is stabilized and the corneal endothelium is protected with viscoelastic or air. A lens glide may be inserted across the anterior chamber into the distal angle to protect the pupil from the advancing IOL haptic. The surgeon then inserts the IOL, placing its leading haptic into the angle while observing the iris for any indication of tuck. As the IOL is held against the distal angle, the glide is withdrawn while the intraocular lens is stabilized with forceps, and the posterior lip of the wound is gently retracted to allow placement of the trailing haptic in the angle. Visual inspection should confirm the proper insertion of the trailing haptic. The surgeon can adjust IOL position by using a hook to flex the optic toward either angle for repositioning.

The pupil will peak toward areas of iris tuck, and the IOL should be repositioned until the pupil is round and the optic is centered. Light indentation of the sclera axial to the lens position should flex the IOL without significant decentration of the optic, movement of the pupil, or rotation of the lens. The viscoelastic is aspirated and the chamber depth is adjusted with balanced salt solution.

Secondary IOL implantation

When spectacles or contact lenses are unsatisfactory for correction of aphakia, secondary IOL implantation is indicated. The type of cataract surgery performed and the general condition of the anterior segment determine the appropriate style and technique of lens implantation. Specific contraindications for primary IOL implantation apply to secondary procedures as well. Secondary procedures cause additional endothelial cell loss and inflammation, thus adding to the risk of corneal decompensation, cystoid macular edema, and secondary glaucoma.

The pupil is dilated for secondary posterior chamber implantation, but it is constricted with preoperative miotic eyedrops for secondary angle-supported IOL implantation. Factors that influence selection of a wound site (superior versus temporal) include preexisting astigmatism, iris anatomy, conjunctival scarring, and corneal vascularization. Anterior vitrectomy may be needed to remove any vitreous incarcerated in the wound or adherent to the iris. Synechiae that will interfere with the positioning of the IOL should be dissected. A lens glide may be useful during insertion of anterior or posterior IOLs, and the anterior chamber depth is generally stabilized with viscoelastic. The positioning of secondary IOLs is similar to that described for primary lenses but may be more difficult because of scarring from the cataract surgery.

Contraindications

Intraocular lenses should not be routinely implanted in eyes with uncontrolled active uveitis because of possible proliferative or adhesive reaction to the lens, with cyclitic or pupillary membrane formation. Fuchs uveitis is an exception in that IOLs may be implanted safely and successfully, although the risk of severe postoperative glaucoma must be considered if this condition is present.

The surgeon must determine whether the support structures within the eye are adequate to maintain centration and stability of the IOL for the type of lens fixation anticipated. When capsular support cannot be reasonably ensured, alternative methods of securing a posterior chamber IOL (eg, iris or transscleral suture fixation) or an angle-supported IOL should be used. Where iris or angle support is inadequate for an anterior chamber lens, a sutured posterior chamber lens may provide an alternative. The additional risk of either alternative should be considered.

Although proliferative diabetic retinopathy and other retinal disorders were formerly considered relative contraindications, prospective studies have shown that these conditions are not adversely affected by posterior chamber IOL implantation that maintains an intact posterior capsule.

Ford JG, Karp CL. *Cataract Surgery and Intraocular Lenses: A 21st-Century Perspective.* 2nd ed. Ophthalmology Monograph 7. San Francisco: American Academy of Ophthalmology; 2001.

Intraocular Lens Implantation in Children

No intraocular lens has received premarket approval from the Food and Drug Administration (FDA) as safe and effective for use in children. Therefore, use of an IOL in a child is considered investigational. The FDA currently recognizes the following 3 mechanisms under which an IOL may be implanted in a child:

- A physician may become a clinical investigator for an IOL manufacturer that has received FDA approval for an investigational device exemption (IDE) to study the use of IOLs in children. Implantation in children under an IDE pediatric study requires institutional review board (IRB) approval.
- IOL manufacturers that do not have an ongoing pediatric IDE will typically request, under their IDE for adults, a waiver of the age indication. Implantation in children under an IDE adult study waiver requires IRB approval.
- A physician may decide to implant an approved lens in a child under the good medical practice rule, which states that good medical practice and patient interests require physicians to use commercially available drugs, devices, and biologics according to their best knowledge and judgment. A physician who uses a product in the practice of medicine for an indication not in the approved labeling has the responsibility to be well informed about the product and to base its use on firm scientific evidence. This usage does not require an IDE or review by an IRB, unless such review is otherwise needed.

Indications

The primary indication for IOL implantation in children is the optical correction of aphakia. Other alternatives for aphakic correction are spectacle lenses and contact lenses. Specific characteristics of the child's visual system—such as growth of the eye and change in refractive error over time, the risk of amblyopia, and an enhanced inflammatory response to cataract surgery—add complexities to the decision whether to implant an IOL in a child's eye.

A growing number of clinical case series support the safety and efficacy of implanting IOLs in the eyes of older children. Implantation of IOLs in children under the age of 2 remains controversial; prospective clinical trials of IOL implantation in children under 2 are under way to provide more information about the safety and efficacy of IOLs in this population.

Contraindications

IOL implantation is relatively contraindicated in eyes with microcornea, sclerocornea, microphthalmos, nanophthalmos, corneal endothelial dystrophy, rubella cataract, significant iris abnormality, uncontrolled glaucoma, persistent fetal vasculature (PFV), proliferative diabetic retinopathy, or uveitis.

Procedure

Ideally, lens power calculations are made using A-scan ultrasonography, which may have to be performed under general anesthesia at the time of surgery. Some surgeons select an IOL power with a refractive goal of emmetropia in patients over 4 years of age, whereas others aim for hyperopia of varying amounts to allow for growth of the eye and resultant refractive power changes. The ideal postoperative refraction for the child's growing eye is the subject of ongoing study.

PMMA lenses have the longest record of biocompatibility and are considered the safest material to use in the pediatric age group; a 1-piece design is preferred. Recently, there has been increasing use of foldable acrylic lenses in pediatric cataract surgery.

Capsular fixation is preferable to fixation in the ciliary sulcus. Because posterior capsular opacification commonly occurs after cataract surgery in children, a large posterior capsular opening is made and limited anterior vitrectomy is performed in young children at the time of the cataract surgery. Alternatively, subsequent Nd:YAG capsulotomy can be performed on many cooperative children after about the age of 6 years.

Postoperative Course

Infants and young children may require a more aggressive postoperative course of topical corticosteroids to reduce inflammatory reaction to surgery. Cycloplegia with cyclopentolate or atropine drops for about 1 month postoperatively is advised. Rapid visual rehabilitation with early refraction and amblyopia therapy is essential. As with other forms of pediatric cataract surgery, the key to success is aggressive amblyopia therapy. (See also BCSC Section 6, *Pediatric Ophthalmology and Strabismus.*)

> Wilson ME. Management of aphakia in children. *Focal Points: Clinical Modules for Ophthalmologists.* San Francisco: American Academy of Ophthalmology; 1999, module 1.

Viscoelastics

Viscoelastic materials protect the corneal endothelium and epithelium from mechanical trauma and maintain an intraocular space, such as the anterior or vitreous chamber, for the period that an incision is open. The introduction of viscoelastic agents for use in intraocular procedures has significantly decreased endothelial cell damage during intraoperative manipulations. The term *viscosurgery* has been used to designate procedures and manipulations performed with viscoelastic substances.

> Lane SS, Lindstrom RL. Viscoelastic agents: formulation, clinical applications, and complications. In: Steinert RF, ed. *Cataract Surgery: Technique, Complications, and Management.* Philadelphia: Saunders; 1995:37–45.

Physical Properties

The physical properties of viscoelastic substances are the result of chain length and molecular interactions within chains and between chains. Important characteristics in describing viscoelastic materials are

- viscoelasticity
- viscosity
- pseudoplasticity
- surface tension
- cohesiveness or dispersiveness

Viscoelasticity

The term *viscoelasticity* means that the substance reacts as an elastic compound or gel when energy is transmitted at a high frequency. At low-frequency energy or with slow impact, the substance reacts primarily as a viscous compound. This mutability means that a viscoelastic material can be slowly introduced into the eye with a 27-gauge cannula and yet can maintain the intraocular space even if the incision is open while manipulations occur in the anterior chamber. The degree of elasticity increases with increasing molecular weight and chain length.

Viscosity

The term *viscosity* describes a resistance to flow or shear force. The higher the molecular weight, the more the compound resists flow. A compound with high viscosity holds its shape better than a compound with low viscosity. The viscosity of a viscoelastic substance at rest is a function of concentration, molecular weight, and the size of the flexible molecules in the material.

Pseudoplasticity

Pseudoplasticity is the ability of the solution to transform under pressure from a gel to a liquidlike substance. In clinical terms, a 0 shear force viscoelastic substance is a lubricant and coats tissues well, but under the influence of stress, it becomes an elastic molecular system.

Surface tension

Surface tension is the coating ability of a viscoelastic material. Lower surface tension provides better coating and a low contact angle.

Cohesive versus dispersive

Cohesive and *dispersive* describe the general behavior of the agent. *Cohesive* viscoelastics adhere to themselves and are generally high-molecular-weight agents with high surface tensions and high pseudoplasticity. *Dispersive* agents, conversely, are substances with little tendency for self-adherence, with generally low molecular weights and good coating abilities (low surface tension). Practically speaking, cohesive agents tend to be easily aspirated and are rapidly removed from the eye. For most applications in cataract surgery, these cohesive characteristics are beneficial. However, in the setting of a posterior capsular rupture, a dispersive viscoelastic is the agent of choice because this material, especially if high in viscosity, will tamponade the vitreous to the posterior capsule and will tend not to be aspirated from the eye during cortical cleanup. In contrast, cohesive agents are preferable when space needs to be maintained, such as during capsulorrhexis. Examples of cohesive agents include Healon, Amvisc, and Provisc. Examples of dispersive agents are Viscoat and Vitrax.

Desired Properties of Viscoelastics

The most important properties of viscoelastic materials are the following:

- maintains space
- spreads and protects tissues
- coats tissues and instruments
- is nontoxic
- is noninflammatory
- is optically clear but visible
- has neutral effect on IOP
- protects the endothelium

Space maintenance

The ability to maintain the anterior chamber for a considerable period, even in the presence of an open incision, is attributable to the rheologic properties of viscosity and elasticity. The higher the viscosity, the better the viscoelastic substance is able to maintain the anterior chamber at rest. The viscous nature of materials that resist a tendency toward flow enables them to retain their shape and volume.

Tissue spreading and protection

In anterior segment surgery, maintaining adequate anterior chamber depth during intraocular manipulations is a significant factor in protecting the corneal endothelium. A viscoelastic agent provides protection in a number of ways: cushioning the endothelium from compression and shear forces, coating the endothelium, and providing space for manipulation between the endothelium and instrument or IOL. A thick layer of high-viscosity agent does not allow an instrument or implant to get close enough to the endothelium to cause damage.

Coating

Studies have shown that sodium hyaluronate, chondroitin sulfate, or hydroxypropyl methylcellulose (HPMC) used to coat an IOL can prevent endothelial cell loss that would otherwise result from abrasion. Thin layers of an intermediate-viscosity agent protect the corneal endothelium as well as high-viscosity agents do. Combined chondroitin sulfate/sodium hyaluronate materials have a lower contact angle and surface tension than sodium hyaluronate. As a result, these materials coat instruments, implants, and intraocular tissue very well. However, the physical properties of lower surface tension and lower contact angle prevent the easy aspiration or irrigation of this material.

Other properties

All available viscoelastic materials are nontoxic, noninflammatory, and optically clear. Fluorescein-colored viscoelastic materials were designed to help the surgeon to identify the viscoelastic within the eye and to ensure that it is completely removed. No evidence at present suggests that viscoelastic agents possess any qualities that are nurturing to the endothelium.

Viscoelastic Substances

Sodium hyaluronate is a biopolymer that occurs in many connective tissues throughout the body. It has a high molecular weight (2.5 million daltons) and a low protein content and carries a single negative charge for the disaccharide unit. Hyaluronate has a half-life of approximately 1 day in the aqueous and a half-life of 3 days in the vitreous.

Chondroitin sulfate is a viscoelastic biopolymer similar to hyaluronate acid but possessing a sulfated group in a double negative charge. Chondroitin sulfate is commonly obtained from shark cartilage.

Hydroxypropyl methylcellulose (HPMC) does not occur naturally in animal tissues but is widely distributed in plant fibers such as cotton and wood. The structure of the commercial product is a cellulose polymer modified by the addition of hydroxypropyl and methyl groups to increase the hydrophilic propensity of the material. Methylcellulose is a nonphysiologic compound that does not appear to be metabolized intraocularly. It is eventually eliminated in the aqueous but can be easily irrigated from the eye.

Polyacrylamide (PA) is a synthetically produced polymer similar to hyaluronate acid. It is a linear, long-chain molecule that is nontoxic, requires no refrigeration, and is inert inside the eye. It is rapidly cleared from the anterior chamber and, because of its stability, does not degrade.

The specific characteristics of commercially available viscoelastic substances are listed in Table 8-2.

Outcomes of Cataract Surgery

Contemporary cataract surgery has an excellent success rate, both in terms of improving visual acuity and enhancing subjective visual function. More than 90% of otherwise healthy eyes achieve a best-corrected postoperative visual acuity of 20/40 or better. The rate of achieving a postoperative acuity of 20/40 or better for all eyes has been reported to be 85%–89%; eyes with comorbid conditions such as diabetic retinopathy, glaucoma, and age-related macular degeneration are included.

Visual acuity is but one measure of the functional success of cataract surgery. Research tools have been developed to assess how cataract progression and cataract surgery affect visual function. One of these, the VF-14 instrument, is a questionnaire administered to patients to measure functional impairment related to vision before and after cataract surgery. Another research tool, the Activities of Daily Vision Scale (ADVS), is a measure of vision-specific functional status.

Prospective studies using these tools show that patients who undergo cataract surgery have significant improvement in many quality-of-life parameters, including community and home activities, mental health, driving, and life satisfaction. Among patients with bilateral cataracts, the quality of life improves after cataract surgery on both the first and second eyes. Restoration of binocular vision appears to provide an additional benefit.

In the typical postoperative regimen, the patient is examined 1 day, 1 week, about 1 month, and about 3 months after cataract surgery. More frequent examinations are indicated if unusual clinical findings are noted or if complications occur. During the post-

Table 8-2 **Physical Properties of Viscoelastic Substances**

	Healon (Sodium hyaluronate 1%)	Healon GV (Sodium hyaluronate 1.4%)	Amvisc (Sodium hyaluronate 1.2%)	Amvisc Plus (Sodium hyaluronate 1.6%)	Chondroitin Sulfate (Generic)	Viscoat (Chondroitin sulfate 4%/sodium hyaluronate 3%)	Occucoat (Hydroxypropyl methylcellulose 2%)	Vitrax (Sodium hyaluronate 3%)	Provisc (Sodium hyaluronate 1%)
Resting viscosity (cps)*	>200,000	2,000,000	100,000	102,000	17,000 at 50%	41,000	†	40,000	†
Dynamic viscosity (cps)‡	40,000–64,000	80,000	40,000	55,000	30 at 20%	40,000	4000	30,000	39,000
Color	Clear	Clear	Clear	Clear	Yellow	Clear	Clear	Clear	Clear
Pseudo-plasticity	+++	++++	+++	+++	No	++	+	+++	+++
Contact angle	60°	†	60°	†	†	52°	50°	†	†

* At shear rate of zero. Data from Arshinoff S. Personal communication.
† Not available.
‡ At shear rate of 2/s, 25°C.
Pseudoplasticity key: + = slight; ++ = fair; +++ = good; ++++ = excellent.

(Adapted with permission from Steinert RF, ed. *Cataract Surgery: Techniques, Complications, and Management.* Philadelphia: WB Saunders Co; 1995.)

operative examinations, the ophthalmologist evaluates the patient's visual acuity and intraocular pressure and performs a slit-lamp examination of the anterior segment. An ophthalmoscopic examination is also advisable during the postoperative period. Counseling and patient education are provided.

Variability in the refractive state of the eye is a normal postoperative finding as wound healing occurs. If sutures are used, they may be cut or removed to reduce surgically induced astigmatism. Refractive error usually stabilizes within 6–12 weeks after surgery, and optical correction can be prescribed at that time. Although refractive stability is achieved more rapidly after small-incision cataract surgery (with or without sutures), the visual outcome at 3 months is comparable.

Complication rates for cataract surgery are low. In a meta-analysis of 90 published studies of cataract surgery outcomes, less than 0.5% of eyes developed endophthalmitis or bullous keratopathy; less than 1% developed retinal detachment; and less than 2% developed dislocation or malposition of the IOL, elevated IOP, or clinically apparent cystoid macular edema. Opacification of the posterior lens capsule is a more common, but less serious, complication. The incidence rate of this complication varies with different studies and depends in part on whether the endpoint is *clinically significant* capsular opacification or *any* detectable opacification. In a meta-analysis of pooled clinical studies, clinically significant opacification of the posterior lens capsule occurred in 19% of eyes over time. In a quantitative study of capsular opacification, the incidence of this complication ranged from 10% to 56% of eyes 3 years after surgery and varied with the type of intraocular lens implant material.

Contemporary cataract surgery is remarkably successful in improving sight and restoring visual function to patients. However, complications can occur, and the operation should not be regarded as a "risk-free" procedure. Chapter 9 discusses the complications of cataract surgery in detail.

Brenner MH, Curbow B, Javitt JC, et al. Vision change and quality of life in the elderly. Response to cataract surgery and treatment of other chronic ocular conditions. *Arch Ophthalmol.* 1993;111:680–685.

Javitt JC, Brenner MH, Curbow B, et al. Outcomes of cataract surgery. Improvement in visual acuity and subjective visual function after surgery in the first, second, and both eyes. *Arch Ophthalmol.* 1993;111:686–691.

Mangione CM, Phillips RS, Lawrence MG, et al. Improved visual function and attenuation of declines in health-related quality of life after cataract extraction. *Arch Ophthalmol.* 1994;112:1419–1425.

Powe NR, Schein OD, Gieser SC, et al. Synthesis of the literature on visual acuity and complications following cataract extraction with intraocular lens implantation. Cataract Patient Outcome Research Team. *Arch Ophthalmol.* 1994;112:239–252. [Note: Published erratum appears in *Arch Ophthalmol.* 1994;112:889.]

Steinberg EP, Tielsch JM, Schein OD, et al. National study of cataract surgery outcomes. Variation in 4-month postoperative outcomes as reflected in multiple outcome measures. *Ophthalmology.* 1994;101:1131–1141.

Steinert RF, Brint SF, White SM, et al. Astigmatism after small incision cataract surgery. A postoperative, randomized, multicenter comparison of 4- and 6.5-mm incisions. *Ophthalmology.* 1991;98:417–424. [Note: Published erratum appears in *Ophthalmology.* 1997;104:1370.]

CHAPTER 9

Complications of Cataract Surgery

Complications of cataract surgery are varied in timing as well as scope. They may occur intraoperatively or in the immediate or late postoperative period (Table 9-1). Therefore, it is necessary to observe the postoperative cataract patient at periodic intervals. A typical postoperative regimen consists of examining the patient 1 day, 1 week, about 1 month, and 3 months following cataract surgery. In case of complications or unusual clinical findings, more frequent examinations are indicated.

Jaffe NS, Jaffe MS, Jaffe GF. *Cataract Surgery and Its Complications.* 6th ed. St Louis: Mosby; 1997.

Krupin T, Kolker AE, eds. *Atlas of Complications in Ophthalmic Surgery.* London: Mosby–Year Book Europe, Ltd; 1993.

Shallow or Flat Anterior Chamber

Intraoperative

The anterior chamber may become shallow during ECCE or phacoemulsification because of an inadequate infusion of balanced salt solution into the anterior chamber, leakage through an oversized wound, external pressure on the globe, or positive vitreous pressure. If the reason for loss of normal chamber depth is not apparent, the surgeon should first raise the infusion bottle height and then check the wound. If the wound is too large, and a significant volume of irrigation fluid flows out of the anterior chamber, a suture placed across the wound to reduce its size will help keep the chamber formed. External pressure on the globe can be relieved by readjusting the surgical drapes or eyelid speculum. Positive vitreous pressure occurs more commonly in obese, bull-necked patients; in those with pulmonary disease such as chronic obstructive pulmonary disease (COPD); and in anxious patients or those with full bladders who perform a Valsalva maneuver. Placing obese patients in reverse Trendelenburg position may be useful. Intravenous mannitol can often reduce the elevated vitreous pressure and allow the case to continue uneventfully.

If the reason for the loss of anterior chamber depth is still unknown, the surgeon should check the red reflex to evaluate the possibility of a suprachoroidal hemorrhage or effusion. Often it is necessary to examine the fundus with an indirect ophthalmoscope to confirm the diagnosis of a suprachoroidal hemorrhage or effusion. If a hemorrhage or effusion is significant, the incisions should be closed and the case postponed until the pressure has decreased.

Table 9-1 **Proportion of Eyes Experiencing Complications Following Cataract Surgery and Intraocular Lens Implantation**

Complication	No. of Studies	Range of Complications Results (% of Eyes)	Total No. of Eyes	Pooled Result (% of Eyes)*
Major, early				
Endophthalmitis	16	0–1.9	30,656	0.13 (0.06–0.17)
Major, late				
Bullous keratopathy	27	0–6.0	15,971	0.3 (0.2–0.4)
Malposition/ dislocation of IOLs	40	0–7.8	17,944	1.1 (0.9–1.2)
Clinical cystoid macular edema	43	0–7.6	20,671	1.4 (1.2–1.6)**
Retinal detachment	42	0–2.0	33,603	0.7 (0.6–0.8)
Other, early				
Wound gape/iris prolapse	17	0–3.0	7,499	0.6 (0.4–0.8)
Anterior chamber hemorrhage	19	0–4.0	7,765	0.5 (0.4–0.7)
Hypopyon	10	0–2.0	3,864	0.2 (0.1–0.2)
Iris trauma	8	0–9.1	5,147	1.3 (1.0–1.6)
Zonular/posterior capsule rupture	38	0–9.9	19,052	3.1 (2.9–3.4)
Vitreous loss	26	0–4.0	14,622	0.8 (0.6–1.0)**
Vitreous hemorrhage	5	0–8.0	4,386	0.3 (0.2–0.5)
Choroidal hemorrhage	3	0–2.0	3,638	0.3 (0.1–0.5)
Other, late				
Uveitis	30	0–13.3	11,339	1.8 (1.5–2.1)**
Increased IOP (closed angle)	11	0–1.6	4,391	0.2 (0.1–0.3)
Increased IOP (open angle)	34	0–19.7	11,376	1.2 (1.0–1.4)
Posterior capsular opacification	41	0.7–47.6	14,677	19.7 (19.1–20.3)

Note: This table is based on a synthesis of the literature and does not account for variation in follow-up intervals.
* Pooled result and 95% confidence interval (CI) weighted by sample size of studies.
** Pooled result and 95% CI weighted by quality score and sample size.

(Reprinted from *Cataract in the Adult Eye.* Preferred Practice Patterns. San Francisco: American Academy of Ophthalmology; 1996. Original source: Powe NR, Schein OD, Gieser SC, et al. Synthesis of the literature on visual acuity and complications following cataract extraction with intraocular lens implantation. *Arch Ophthalmol.* 1994;112:239–252.)

Posterior infusion syndrome

In rare cases, the fluid infused into the anterior chamber may be misdirected into the vitreous cavity, causing an increase in the vitreous volume, with subsequent forward displacement of the lens and shallowing of the anterior chamber. The fluid may accumulate in the retrolenticular space or dissect posteriorly along the vitreoretinal interface. This complication is most likely to occur during hydrodissection, when fluid is forcefully injected into the capsular bag. A shallow anterior chamber resulting from posterior infusion syndrome may indicate loss of integrity of the capsular bag, damaged zonular fibers, or misplacement of the irrigating tip. If gentle posterior pressure on the lens does not alleviate the situation, infusing intravenous mannitol and waiting several minutes may allow the anterior chamber to deepen. In addition, the surgeon can insert a 19-gauge needle through the pars plana into the retrolenticular space and gently aspirate to try to remove the fluid and deepen the anterior chamber. Care must be exercised in placing the needle to avoid a retinal tear or detachment. Alternatively, a pars plana vitrectomy may be performed.

Postoperative

A flat anterior chamber during the postoperative period may cause permanent damage to ocular structures. Prolonged apposition of the iris to angle structures can cause permanent peripheral anterior synechiae and chronic angle-closure glaucoma. Following either ICCE or ECCE, iridovitreal or iridocapsular synechiae can also lead to pupillary block. Corneal contact with either vitreous or an IOL can result in endothelial cell loss and chronic corneal edema.

Flat anterior chambers can be classified according to etiology and level of intraocular pressure. Classification by etiology includes the following:

- wound leak
- choroidal detachment
- pupillary block
- ciliary block
- suprachoroidal hemorrhage

Cases associated with ocular hypotension (IOP below 10 mm Hg) are usually secondary to leakage of aqueous at the wound site or choroidal detachment. Patients may be asymptomatic, especially if a wound leak is followed by iris incarceration, allowing reformation of the anterior chamber. Even without iris incarceration, slow or intermittent wound leaks may coexist with a formed anterior chamber. Careful comparison of chamber depth with that of the fellow eye may be helpful in identifying these cases.

To detect an area of wound leakage, it is usually sufficient to paint the surface of the incision with a fluorescein strip or instill 1 or 2 drops of 2% fluorescein, and then examine the entire incision with the cobalt blue filter on the slit lamp (Seidel test). Aqueous dilution of fluorescein at the site of wound leakage will produce a contrasting area of green stain. Occasionally, aqueous flow is so slight that gentle pressure on the globe is necessary to confirm the site of leakage.

The physician managing a wound leak can consider several options:

- Some eyes with wound leaks may respond within hours to cycloplegia and pressure patching.
- Carbonic anhydrase inhibitors and topical beta blockers may decrease aqueous flow through the wound.
- Avoiding the use of steroids enhances local wound reaction to facilitate spontaneous closure.

- Therapeutic soft contact lenses have been successful in reducing aqueous flow through the wound.
- Tissue adhesive may seal the wound and allow it to heal in selected cases.

These methods are appropriate both for the management of minor wound leaks with adequate and secure wound apposition and as temporary measures until more secure wound closure can be accomplished surgically. Patients may develop an associated cilio-choroidal detachment that resolves spontaneously after wound closure. Surgical exploration, with re-formation of the anterior chamber and wound repair, is indicated if no improvement occurs within 24–48 hours, if obvious wound separation is present, if the iris is prolapsed out of the wound, or if intraocular structures such as the IOL are in contact with the corneal endothelium.

Late *hypotony* without obvious wound leak is uncommon after cataract surgery. It may result from retinal detachment, cyclodialysis, filtering bleb formation, or persistent uveitis.

Cases of a shallow anterior chamber with normal or high IOP are usually the result of pupillary block, ciliary block, or suprachoroidal hemorrhage. Pupillary block that occurs in the early postoperative period may follow a resolved wound leak. Postoperative uveitis with iridovitreal or iridocapsular synechiae may cause relatively late pupillary block. Failure to perform a peripheral iridectomy after placement of an anterior chamber IOL may also be associated with early or late postoperative pupillary block. If initial attempts at pupillary dilation fail to deepen the anterior chamber and lower the pressure, a laser peripheral iridotomy is usually effective.

Aqueous sequestration within the vitreous body may be the cause of ciliary block glaucoma, with a flat anterior chamber and high IOP that is unresponsive to medical therapy or peripheral iridectomy. Vitrectomy is the preferred treatment for this rare condition.

Corneal Edema

Stromal and Epithelial Edema

Stromal and/or epithelial edema may occur in the immediate postoperative period. The incidence is higher in eyes with preexisting corneal endothelial dysfunction. Edema is most often caused by a combination of mechanical trauma, prolonged intraocular irrigation, inflammation, and elevated IOP, resulting in acute endothelial decompensation with an increase in corneal thickness. It generally resolves completely within 4–6 weeks following surgery. If epithelial edema is present in the face of a compact stroma immediately after surgery, it is likely due to elevated IOP with intact endothelium. Decreasing IOP via aqueous release from the paracentesis site often results in immediate resolution of epithelial edema in these cases. As a rule, if the corneal periphery is clear, the corneal edema will usually resolve with time. Corneal edema persisting after 3 months usually does not clear and may require penetrating keratoplasty.

Brown-McLean Syndrome

Brown-McLean syndrome, a clinical condition that may occur after cataract surgery, consists of peripheral corneal edema with a clear central cornea. This condition occurs most frequently following intracapsular cataract surgery, but it has also been reported following extracapsular and phacoemulsification surgery. The edema typically starts inferiorly and progresses circumferentially but spares the central cornea. Central corneal guttae (cornea guttata) frequently appear, and punctate brown pigment often underlies the edematous areas. In rare cases, Brown-McLean syndrome progresses to clinically significant central corneal edema. The etiology of this syndrome is unknown.

Brown SI, McLean JM. Peripheral corneal edema after cataract extraction. A new clinical entity. *Trans Am Acad Ophthalmol Otolaryngol.* 1969;73:465–470.

Gothard TW, Hardten DR, Lane SS, et al. Clinical findings in Brown-McLean syndrome. *Am J Ophthalmol.* 1993;115:729–737.

Vitreocorneal Adherence and Persistent Corneal Edema

Vitreocorneal adherence and persistent corneal edema can occur early or late after uncomplicated ICCE or after complicated ECCE. A vitrectomy may be indicated if corneal thickening or edema develops. In more advanced cases with prolonged corneal edema, penetrating keratoplasty combined with vitrectomy may be indicated.

Corneal Complications of Phacoemulsification

During phacoemulsification, heat may be transferred from the probe to the cornea. A wound that is too tight to allow adequate irrigation fluid flow along the vibrating probe or the occlusion of irrigation or aspiration tubing by viscoelastic or lens material can be the cause of such heat transfer. Higher aspiration flow rates and vacuum, lower ultrasound energy levels, and use of cohesive viscoelastics during portions of the procedure when occlusion is likely to occur, may reduce the risk of this complication. If the cornea clouds during the phacoemulsification procedure and reduces the visibility of the nucleus, the surgeon can convert to a nuclear expression technique if necessary.

When corneal wound burns occur, the heat causes contraction of the corneal collagen with subsequent distortion of the wound. If the wound distortion is significant, wound gape may occur with associated wound leak. These types of wounds will not be self-sealing and require suturing for adequate closure. The first priority is closing the wound with sutures, even if this maneuver induces astigmatism. After approximately 6 weeks, the sutures can be selectively removed based on keratometry or corneal topography and an assessment of the integrity of the wound.

Holding the phaco tip too close to the corneal endothelium during surgery allows the ultrasonic energy to injure and cause loss of the endothelial cells. Performing phacoemulsification or allowing lens fragments to circulate in the anterior chamber without adequate viscoelastic protection can contribute to endothelial cell loss. These cases may demonstrate corneal edema on the first postoperative day, or its appearance may be delayed months to years following surgery.

Nuclear fragments in contact with the endothelium may cause corneal edema. Small retained nuclear fragments in the anterior chamber angle may contribute to focal corneal edema. Removing retained nuclear material may allow for the corneal edema to resolve.

Detachment of Descemet's Membrane

Detachment of Descemet's membrane results in stromal swelling and epithelial bullae localized in the area of detachment. This complication can occur when an instrument or IOL is introduced through the cataract incision or when fluid is inadvertently injected between Descemet's membrane and the corneal stroma. Small detachments may resolve spontaneously. Otherwise, they may be reattached with air or expansile gas [eg, sulfur hexafluoride (SF_6) or perfluoropropane (C_3F_8)] tamponade in the anterior chamber. Larger detachments can be sutured back into place. Gas may help to position the detached area of Descemet's membrane prior to suture placement. Viscoelastic can facilitate chamber maintenance during the procedure, but great care must be taken not to introduce it between Descemet's membrane and corneal stroma. One or more 10–0 nylon sutures armed with long, curved cutting needles on both ends may be used. The needles are first passed through the incision or peripheral cornea distant to the area of Descemet's detachment. The needles are then passed from the anterior chamber and through the detached area of Descemet's membrane, stroma, and epithelium. The ends are tied on the external surface of the cornea, and the knots are buried.

Toxic Solutions

Certain solutions, either irrigated or inadvertently injected into the anterior chamber, can be toxic to the corneal endothelium and cause temporary or permanent corneal edema. Subconjunctival antibiotic injections have been reported to enter the anterior chamber through scleral tunnel incisions that act as 1-way valves. Skin cleansers containing chlorhexidine gluconate (eg, Hibiclens) have been reported to cause irreversible corneal edema and opacification if they inadvertently come into contact with the corneal surface. Preservatives present in prediluted epinephrine (1:10,000) added to irrigating solutions have been implicated in corneal decompensation. Unpreserved 1:1000 epinephrine is preferred. Substitution of sterile water for balanced salt solution, intraocular use of preserved medications, or inadvertent intraocular injection of residual toxic materials, which may be present in reusable cannulas or irrigation tubing, may cause severe endothelial damage.

Monson MC, Mamalis N, Olson RJ. Toxic anterior segment inflammation following cataract surgery. *J Cataract Refract Surg.* 1992;18:184–189.

Hejny C, Edelhauser HF. Surgical pharmacology: intraocular solutions and drugs used for cataract surgery. In: Buratto L, Werner L, Zanini M, et al, eds. *Phacoemulsification: Principles and Techniques.* 2nd ed. Thorofare, NJ: Slack; 2003:ch 12.

Hemorrhage

A recent large prospective cohort study was unable to demonstrate an increased risk of hemorrhagic complications in patients on anticoagulant or antiplatelet therapy during cataract surgery. In addition, no increase in medical complications was observed when such therapy was temporarily discontinued for surgery. This contrasts with earlier reports, which suggested that anticoagulation increases the risk of suprachoroidal effusion and suprachoroidal hemorrhage.

Katz J, Feldman MA, Bass EB, et al. Risks and benefits of anticoagulant and antiplatelet medication use before cataract surgery. *Ophthalmology.* 2003;110:1784–1788.

Retrobulbar Hemorrhage

Retrobulbar hemorrhages are more common with retrobulbar anesthetic injections than with peribulbar injections, and they may vary in intensity. Reports estimate the incidence of significant retrobulbar hemorrhage to be 1%–3%. *Venous* retrobulbar hemorrhages are usually self-limited and tend to spread slowly. They often do not require treatment.

Arterial retrobulbar hemorrhages occur more rapidly and are associated with taut orbital swelling, marked proptosis, elevated intraocular pressure, reduced mobility of the globe, inability to separate the eyelids, and massive ecchymosis of the lids and conjunctiva. This type of retrobulbar hemorrhage causes an increase in orbital volume and associated orbital pressure, which can restrict the vascular supply to the globe. Large orbital vessels may be occluded, or tamponade of the smaller nutrient vessels in the optic nerve may occur, resulting in severe visual loss and subsequent optic atrophy despite the absence of obvious retinal vascular occlusion.

The diagnosis of retrobulbar hemorrhage is often made by observing the rapid onset of lid and conjunctival ecchymosis and tightening of the orbit. It can be confirmed by tonometry revealing elevated intraocular pressure. A simple handheld tonometer kept in a sterile pack in the operating room is ideal for this situation. Direct ophthalmoscopy may reveal pulsation or occlusion of the central retinal artery in severe cases.

Treatment of acute retrobulbar hemorrhage consists of maneuvers to rapidly lower the orbital and intraocular pressure. These maneuvers may include digital massage, intravenous osmotic agents, topical aqueous suppressants, lateral canthotomy and cantholysis, localized conjunctival peritomy (to allow egress of blood), and, occasionally, even anterior chamber paracentesis. Serial tonometry demonstrating a reduction in intraocular pressure will help confirm the success of the treatment. In general, cataract surgery should not be performed when a serious retrobulbar hemorrhage occurs because the risk of iris prolapse or even an expulsive choroidal hemorrhage is far greater than usual. The surgery can be rescheduled for several days later. To reduce the risk of a recurrent retrobulbar hemorrhage, many surgeons would consider using peribulbar, sub-Tenon's, topical, or general anesthesia for the second attempt at surgery.

Cionni R, Osher RH. Retrobulbar hemorrhage. *Ophthalmology.* 1991;98:1153–1155.

Feibel RM. Current concepts in retrobulbar anesthesia. *Surv Ophthalmol.* 1985;30:102–110.

Morgan CM, Schatz H, Vine AK, et al. Ocular complications associated with retrobulbar anesthesia. *Ophthalmology.* 1988;95:660–665.

Suprachoroidal Hemorrhage or Effusion

Suprachoroidal effusion with or without suprachoroidal hemorrhage generally occurs intraoperatively. Secure wound fixation to prevent hypotony can significantly reduce the postoperative risk of this complication. Typically, a forward prolapse of posterior ocular structures including iris and vitreous occurs, generally accompanied by a change in the red reflex. Clinically, suprachoroidal effusion may be difficult to differentiate from suprachoroidal hemorrhage. Both complications are more common in the presence of underlying hypertension, obesity, high myopia, anticoagulation, glaucoma, or chronic ocular inflammation. Fortunately, both complications are much less likely with modern phacoemulsification because of the relatively closed system formed by small-incision, self-sealing wound architecture, and the relatively tight fit of the phaco tip in the wound.

Suprachoroidal effusion may be a precursor of suprachoroidal hemorrhage. Exudation of fluid from choroidal vasculature ultimately tents veins or arteries that supply the choroid after coursing through the sclera. If suprachoroidal hemorrhage occurs in this situation, it is presumably a result of disruption of one or more of these tented blood vessels. Alternatively, suprachoroidal hemorrhage may represent a spontaneous rupture of choroidal vasculature, particularly in patients with underlying systemic vascular disease.

Expulsive Suprachoroidal Hemorrhage

Expulsive suprachoroidal hemorrhage, a rare but serious problem, generally occurs intraoperatively. It requires immediate action. This condition usually presents as a sudden increase in IOP accompanied by darkening of the red reflex; wound gape; iris prolapse; expulsion of the lens, vitreous, and bright red blood; or sudden onset of pain. The instant this condition is recognized, the wound must be closed with sutures or digital pressure. Posterior sclerotomies allow the escape of suprachoroidal blood, which may help to decompress the globe; allow the repositioning of prolapsed intraocular tissue; and facilitate permanent closure of the cataract incision. If the incision can be closed without posterior sclerotomies, more rapid tamponade of the bleeding vessel is achieved. There is no clear consensus on whether visual outcomes are superior with or without posterior sclerotomies.

Treatment of both suprachoroidal and expulsive suprachoroidal hemorrhage consists of rapid wound closure. Subsequent elevation of IOP will tamponade the bleeding. Having closed the globe, the surgeon may wish to drain the suprachoroidal blood by performing a sclerotomy in one or more quadrants, 5–7 mm posterior to the limbus, if a hemorrhagic component can be seen. If the involved quadrants can't be readily identified, posterior sclerotomies can empirically be placed in the inferotemporal quadrant. If this attempt fails to adequately drain the suprachoroidal hemorrhage, additional sclerotomies can be placed in the other quadrants. The sclerotomy can be created with either a blade or a small (Elliot) trephine. Hemorrhagic fluid is drained, while the elevated IOP serves both to stop bleeding and to expel suprachoroidal blood. Once optimal clearance of blood from the suprachoroidal space has occurred, the surgeon may wish to leave the sclerotomies open to allow further drainage postoperatively. In addition, the surgeon may consider repeating the drainage procedure 7 days or more after an expulsive hemorrhage in case of residual suprachoroidal blood that could threaten ocular integrity or visual acuity. These procedures may lower dangerously elevated IOPs and restore appropriate anatomic relationships within the eye, but they carry some risk that bleeding will recur. Some surgeons prefer to close the wound and refer the patient to a vitreoretinal specialist.

Delayed Suprachoroidal Hemorrhage

Less commonly, suprachoroidal hemorrhage may occur in the early postoperative period, presenting with sudden onset of pain, loss of vision, and shallowing of the anterior chamber. If the wound remains intact and the IOP can be controlled medically, limited suprachoroidal hemorrhage may be observed and frequently will resolve spontaneously. If the wound is not intact, surgical wound revision alone may be sufficient to allow the hemorrhage to resolve. Surgical drainage of the suprachoroidal space is indicated with persistent flat anterior chamber, medically uncontrolled glaucoma, adherent (kissing) choroidals, or persistent choroidal detachment. Medical management consists of empiric systemic corticosteroids, topical and oral ocular hypotensive agents, topical cycloplegia, and close observation.

Hyphema

Hyphema in the immediate postoperative period usually originates from the incision or the iris; it is commonly mild and resolves spontaneously. Resolution may take longer if vitreous is mixed with the blood. The two major complications from prolonged hyphema are elevated IOP and corneal blood staining. IOP should be monitored closely and treated in the usual medical fashion, although it may be difficult to control if the blood is mixed with the viscoelastic used during the procedure.

Hyphema that occurs months to years after surgery usually comes from wound vascularization or erosion of vascular tissue by an IOL. Argon laser photocoagulation of the bleeding vessel, often performed through a goniolens, will usually stop the bleeding or prevent rebleeding. To reduce the risk of continued or recurrent bleeding, antiplatelet or anticoagulation therapy may be withheld, if medically possible, until the hyphema resolves.

Retinal Light Toxicity

Prolonged exposure to the illuminating filament of the operating microscope can result in an increased risk of cystoid macular edema or a burn to the retinal pigment epithelium (RPE). This problem is especially serious during cataract surgery, when the filtering effects of the natural lens (cataract) are removed, exposing the vulnerable RPE to unfiltered blue light and near-UV radiation. If the burn occurs in the fovea, visual acuity may be reduced. If the burn is extrafoveal, the patient may complain of a paracentral scotoma. Minimizing retinal exposure to the operating microscope light is the key to avoiding this complication.

Actions to reduce the risk of retinal photic injury include the following:

- Use only the light intensity needed to clearly visualize and perform the surgical procedure.
- Replace lamps with manufacturer-approved products.

- Add a filter to exclude light below 515 nm.
- Use oblique lighting, if possible.
- Use pupillary shields, either built into the microscope or placed on the cornea.
- Minimize direct exposure of the fovea.

Retinal photic injuries from operating microscopes during cataract surgery. FDA Public Health Advisory. Rockville, MD: US Dept Health and Human Services; 1995.

Elevated Intraocular Pressure

A rise in IOP is common following cataract surgery. It is generally mild and self-limited and does not require prolonged antiglaucoma therapy. However, a significant and sustained rise in IOP following cataract surgery may necessitate timely and specific management in several circumstances.

Viscoelastic material such as hyaluronate retained in the eye after cataract surgery is frequently responsible for postoperative IOP elevation. Even when it is removed from the anterior chamber at the conclusion of surgery, viscoelastic material can be sequestered in the posterior chamber or behind the lens implant. Mixtures of chondroitin and hyaluronate have been advocated to reduce the risk of this occurrence; however, even these combinations are associated with elevated IOP in certain patients. IOP elevation usually does not last more than a few days and is amenable to medical treatment. Marked IOP elevation in the early postoperative period may be managed expeditiously by releasing a small amount of aqueous humor with gentle pressure on the posterior lip of a preexisting paracentesis. Preparation of the ocular surface with topical antibiotics or povidone-iodine is desirable. Topical and/or systemic pressure-lowering agents should also be administered, as pressure reduction after aqueous release is short-lived.

Other causes of elevated IOP after cataract surgery include pupillary block, hyphema, ciliary block, endophthalmitis, retained lens material (phacolytic or phacoanaphylactic reactions), iris pigment release, preexisting glaucoma, corticosteroid usage, or peripheral anterior synechiae. The latter may result from a flat anterior chamber in the early postoperative period when the eye is inflamed. It may produce severe secondary glaucoma at a later time. Treating the underlying cause of the IOP elevation should be curative.

Cystoid Macular Edema

Cystoid macular edema (CME) is a common cause of decreased vision after both complicated and uncomplicated cataract surgery (in these cases it is also known as *Irvine-Gass syndrome*). Although its pathogenesis is unknown, the final common pathway appears to be increased perifoveolar capillary permeability, possibly associated with generalized intraocular vascular instability. Associated factors include inflammation with release of prostaglandins, vitreomacular traction, excessive ultraviolet light exposure, posterior capsule rupture, vitreous loss, iris prolapse, and transient or prolonged hypotony.

CME can be recognized by an otherwise unexplained reduction in visual acuity or by the characteristic appearance of the macula on ophthalmoscopy or fluorescein angiography (Fig 9-1) or by ocular coherence tomography (OCT). *Angiographic* CME occurs in 40%–70% of eyes following ICCE and about 1%–19% of eyes following ECCE via nuclear expression or phacoemulsification. Most of the affected patients are visually asymptomatic.

If the diagnosis of *clinical* CME is based on visual loss to the 20/40 level or worse, the incidence is 2%–10% following intracapsular surgery and 1%–2% following extra-capsular surgery with an intact posterior capsule. The risk of clinical CME after phacoe-mulsification with an intact posterior capsule is believed to be even lower. However, patients with *angiographic* CME after phacoemulsification demonstrate significantly lower logMAR visual acuity scores than patients with no CME, even though their Snellen visual acuities remain better than 20/40. The peak incidence occurs 6–10 weeks after surgery. Spontaneous resolution occurs in approximately 95% of uncomplicated cases, usually within 6 months. Rarely, CME may develop many years after ICCE, especially in association with delayed postoperative rupture of the anterior hyaloid face. It is also associated with the use of epinephrine and dipivefrin medications for the treatment of aphakic glaucoma. The prostaglandin analogue latanoprost has also been associated with reversible CME in eyes that have undergone recent intraocular surgery, though a cause-and-effect relationship has not been established. The risk is believed to be greater in the absence of an intact posterior capsule. Other risk factors for CME include poorly con-trolled postoperative inflammation, preexisting epiretinal membrane, diabetes mellitus, and a previous history of CME.

The relationship between IOL implants and both clinical and angiographic CME is not completely understood. Some retrospective studies suggest a higher incidence and later onset, as well as a poorer prognosis, in eyes with iris-supported IOLs. Closed-loop anterior chamber IOLs are associated with a high incidence of uveitis, CME, glaucoma, hyphema, and corneal decompensation. Quiet postoperative eyes with evidence of mal-positioned implants (iris tuck, intermittent corneal touch, pupillary capture, short an-terior chamber lens), as well as eyes with implant-related uveitis, show a higher incidence of chronic CME. The presence of a well-positioned posterior chamber or open-loop

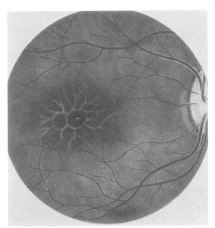
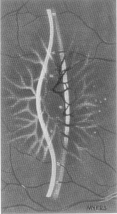

Figure 9-1 Artist's render-ing of cystic spaces in macula associated with cystoid macular edema. *(Reprinted from Gass JD, Norton EW. Cystoid macular edema and papilledema following cataract ex-traction. A fluorescein fundoscopic and angiographic study.* Arch Ophthalmol. *1966;76:647.)*

anterior chamber IOL does not appear to increase the risk of CME. A UV-filtering IOL may reduce the incidence of angiographic CME after cataract surgery.

CME with visual loss occurs more commonly in eyes with surgical complications and in eyes with vitreous adhering to the incision, the iris, or the intraocular lens. The risk of CME can be reduced with pre- and postoperative prophylactic use of topical or systemic indomethacin or topical ketorolac. Because most cases of postoperative CME resolve spontaneously, it is difficult to assess the effect of therapeutic agents. Topical ketorolac 0.5% has been demonstrated to be an effective treatment for chronic CME in a prospective, randomized, controlled clinical trial. Greater improvement in acuity was obtained with a combination of topical ketorolac 0.5% and prednisolone 1% 4 times a day than with either medication alone. If topical medications fail, some surgeons will try sub-Tenon's injections of corticosteroids. There have been anecdotal reports of success with systemic nonsteroidal anti-inflammatory agents, carbonic anhydrase inhibitors, or corticosteroids or with hyperbaric oxygen or intravitreal triamcinolone acetonide (Kenalog). Despite the lack of controlled clinical studies, it is believed that prophylaxis with any one of several topical nonsteroidal anti-inflammatory drops will be of benefit in CME prophylaxis and treatment.

Surgical therapy is indicated when chronic clinical CME fails to respond to medical therapy. Nd:YAG laser treatment or vitrectomy surgery can be used to remove vitreous adhering to the cataract incision, thus relieving vitreomacular traction. This approach has been shown to be of value in patients with chronic CME, especially when medically unresponsive, low-grade uveitis is present. IOL exchange may be helpful if the IOL is malpositioned, has vitreous adherent to it, or contributes to chronic uveitis. Laser grid therapy has been reported only anecdotally in patients with diabetes who have chronic CME. (For further discussion of cystoid macular edema, see BCSC Section 12, *Retina and Vitreous*.)

Conway MD, Canakis C, Livir-Rallatos C, et al. Intravitreal triamcinolone acetonide for refractory chronic pseudophakic cystoid macular edema. *J Cataract Refract Surg*. 2003;29: 27–33.

Flach AJ, Jampol LM, Weinberg D, et al. Improvement in visual acuity in chronic aphakic and pseudophakic cystoid macular edema after treatment with topical 0.5% ketorolac tromethamine. *Am J Ophthalmol*. 1991;112:514–519.

Heier JS, Topping TM, Baumann W, et al. Ketorolac versus prednisolone versus combination therapy in the treatment of acute pseudophakic cystoid macular edema. *Ophthalmology*. 2000;107:2034–2038.

Jaffe GJ. Cystoid macular edema. *Focal Points: Clinical Modules for Ophthalmologists*. 1994, module 11.

Kraff MC, Sanders DR, Jampol LM, et al. Factors affecting pseudophakic cystoid macular edema: five randomized trials. *J Am Intraocul Implant Soc*. 1985;11:380–385.

Ursell PG, Spalton DJ, Whitcup SM, et al. Cystoid macular edema after phacoemulsification: relationship to blood-aqueous barrier damage and visual acuity. *J Cataract Refract Surg*. 1999;25:1492–1497.

Wand M, Shields BM. Cystoid macular edema in the era of ocular hypotensive lipids. *Am J Ophthalmol*. 2002;133:393–397.

Retinal Detachment

Retinal detachment occurs in 2%–3% of eyes following ICCE and in 0.5%–2.0% of eyes following ECCE. The incidence of retinal detachment following phacoemulsification is believed to occur in an even smaller percentage of patients. Retinal detachment occurs most frequently within 6 months of cataract surgery or following posterior capsulotomy (Fig 9-2).

Predisposing factors include axial myopia (greater than 25 mm), lattice degeneration of the retina, a previous retinal tear or detachment in the operated eye, a history of retinal detachment in the fellow eye, and a family history of retinal detachment. The presence of any of these factors should make the surgeon more vigilant in examining the peripheral fundus in these patients before and after surgery and should be considered in the decision to treat asymptomatic retinal breaks preoperatively.

The presence of an intact posterior capsule reduces the incidence of retinal detachment. Conversely, complicated cataract surgery with a broken posterior capsule and vitreous loss increases the postoperative risk of retinal detachment. Evidence suggests that the risk of retinal detachment increases fourfold following Nd:YAG laser posterior capsulotomy. Anecdotal reports have suggested that delaying the Nd:YAG laser posterior capsulotomy may reduce the risk of subsequent retinal detachment. Although there are no prospective, randomized, controlled studies to confirm this belief, delaying capsulotomy for at least 3–6 months after cataract surgery may allow for posterior vitreous separation and thus be less disruptive to the vitreoretinal interface. The successful repair of retinal detachment is not influenced by the presence or absence of either an anterior or a posterior chamber IOL.

Haller JA. Retinal detachment. *Focal Points: Clinical Modules for Ophthalmologists.* San Francisco: American Academy of Ophthalmology; 1998, module 5.

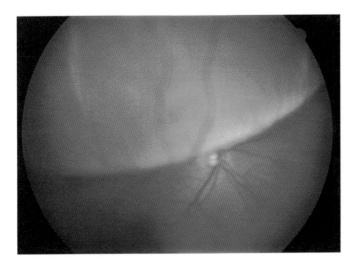

Figure 9-2 Bullous superior rhegmatogenous retinal detachment following extracapsular cataract extraction and posterior chamber lens implantation. *(Reproduced with permission from Wilkinson CP. Retinal complications following cataract surgery. Focal Points: Clinical Modules for Ophthalmologists. San Francisco: American Academy of Ophthalmology; 1992, module 12.)*

Wilkinson CP. Retinal complications following cataract surgery. *Focal Points: Clinical Modules for Ophthalmologists.* San Francisco: American Academy of Ophthalmology; 1992, module 12.

Endophthalmitis

Endophthalmitis may present in an acute form or in a more indolent or chronic form; the latter is associated with organisms of lower pathogenicity. The symptoms of endophthalmitis include mild to severe ocular pain, loss of vision, floaters, and photophobia. The hallmark of endophthalmitis is vitreous inflammation, but other signs include eyelid or periorbital edema, ciliary injection, chemosis, anterior chamber reaction, hypopyon, decreased visual acuity, corneal edema, and retinal hemorrhages (Fig 9-3).

Diagnosis

Acute endophthalmitis typically develops 2–5 days postoperatively and runs a fulminant course. Decreasing vision and increasing pain and inflammation are hallmarks. Early diagnosis is extremely important, as delay of treatment can substantially alter the visual prognosis. *Chronic endophthalmitis,* in contrast, may have its onset weeks or months after surgery. It may be characterized by chronic iritis or granulomatous uveitis and is often associated with decreased visual acuity, little or no pain, and the presence of a sequestrum of the infectious agent within the eye. (See also BCSC Section 9, *Intraocular Inflammation and Uveitis,* and BCSC Section 12, *Retina and Vitreous.*)

Noninfectious (sterile) endophthalmitis is a rare complication of cataract surgery. It is often associated with the introduction of toxic materials into the eye via contaminants on an IOL, inadvertent intracameral injection of a toxin, or a severe inflammatory reaction to retained lens material. The diagnosis of sterile endophthalmitis is made by excluding possible infectious causes by means of appropriate aqueous and vitreous cultures.

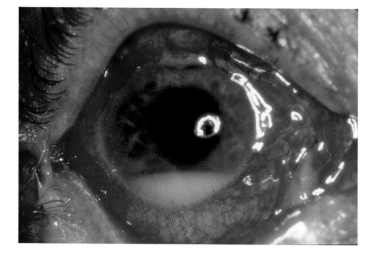

Figure 9-3 Endophthalmitis. *(Photograph courtesy of Karla J. Johns, MD.)*

Treatment

The recommended approach to the diagnosis and management of postoperative endophthalmitis is based on the results of the Endophthalmitis Vitrectomy Study (EVS). In this study, patients were randomized to receive either an immediate 3-port pars plana vitrectomy (VIT) or tap/biopsy of the vitreous (TAP). Patients were further randomized to either receive or not receive intravenous antibiotics. All study patients received a standard antibiotic regimen consisting of 0.4 mg/0.1 mL intravitreal amikacin and 1.0 mg/0.1 mL intravitreal vancomycin, along with subconjunctival injections of 25 mg vancomycin, 100 mg ceftazidime, and 6 mg dexamethasone. Topical antibiotics included 50 mg/mL vancomycin and 14 mg/mL amikacin, which were administered along with topical cycloplegics and corticosteroids. Patients assigned to intravenous antibiotics received ceftazidime and amikacin.

Vitreous cultures were positive in 69% of cases, with gram-positive, coagulase-negative staphylococcus species (especially *Staphylococcus epidermidis*) representing 70% of the positive cultures. Other gram-positive organisms were recovered in about 15% of cases, gram-negative species in 5.9% of cases, and polymicrobial growth in 9.3% of cases.

Final posttreatment visual acuity of 20/40 or better was achieved by 53% of all study patients in the EVS, with 74% attaining 20/100 or better. For all study patients who presented with better than light perception (LP) vision (ie, hand motions or better), the visual results were equal in both groups; there were no benefits with either VIT or TAP in the final visual outcome. Vitrectomy was found to be of benefit only for those patients presenting with LP vision, as VIT patients achieved better visual acuity than TAP patients. No benefit was found with the use of intravenous antibiotics. This result is not surprising given the poor penetration of most intravenous antibiotics into the vitreous cavity.

As soon as endophthalmitis is recognized, assessment of visual acuity will help direct the management decisions. Fortified topical antibiotics may be started if doing so does not delay referral to a vitreoretinal specialist. Immediate 3-port pars plana vitrectomy is indicated when vision has been reduced to light perception, whereas less invasive vitreous biopsy or needle aspiration is adequate when the vision is hand motions or better. Because there are no reliable clinical features to distinguish between gram-positive and gram-negative organisms, the mainstay of treatment for both remains broad-spectrum intravitreal antibiotics. Fortified topical and subconjunctival antibiotics are administered in the period following antibiotic injection into the vitreous, while waiting for culture results. Intravenous antibiotics are of no benefit. Although frequently used because of their theoretical role in reducing inflammation and scarring, the benefit of intravitreal corticosteroids has yet to be demonstrated in a controlled study. Oral fluoroquinolones have been shown to achieve significant levels in the aqueous and vitreous fluids. Although not proven in a controlled study, there may be theoretical benefits to oral fluoroquinolones in the treatment of endophthalmitis.

Doft BH. Managing infectious endophthalmitis: results of the Endophthalmitis Vitrectomy Study. *Focal Points: Clinical Modules for Ophthalmologists.* San Francisco: American Academy of Ophthalmology; 1997, module 3.

A randomized trial of immediate vitrectomy and of intravenous antibiotics for the treatment of postoperative bacterial endophthalmitis. Endophthalmitis Vitrectomy Study Group. *Arch Ophthalmol.* 1995;113:1479–1496.

Macular Infarction

Extensive retinal nonperfusion and macular infarction, clinically similar in appearance to central retinal artery occlusion, may occur after uncomplicated subconjunctival injection of aminoglycosides for endophthalmitis prophylaxis at the conclusion of cataract surgery. This complication appears to be uncommon, but the incidence is unknown. The risk may be greatest with gentamicin, but amikacin and tobramycin can cause a similar clinical picture. There is little evidence that subconjunctival aminoglycoside injection reduces the incidence of post–cataract surgery endophthalmitis, especially in light of the EVS finding that gram-positive organisms are the etiologic agent in 70% of culture-positive cases. Endophthalmitis is treatable, whereas macular infarction is not. Therefore, routine subconjunctival aminoglycoside prophylaxis is no longer recommended at the conclusion of cataract surgery.

Campochiaro PA, Conway BP. Aminoglycoside toxicity—a survey of retinal specialists. *Arch Ophthalmol.* 1991;109:946–950.

Chronic Uveitis

Chronic uveitis following cataract surgery has been reported in association with low-grade bacterial pathogens, including *Propionibacterium acnes* and *S epidermidis*. Uveitis patients may have an unremarkable early postoperative course and lack the classic findings of acute endophthalmitis. Weeks or months after surgery, however, these patients develop chronic uveitis that is variably responsive to topical corticosteroids. This condition is usually associated with granulomatous keratic precipitates and less commonly with hypopyon. A localized focus or sequestrum of infection may occasionally be observed, most often within the remaining lens capsule. Diagnosis requires a high level of clinical suspicion, coupled with examination and cultures of appropriate specimens of aqueous, vitreous, and, where applicable, retained lens material that may harbor a sequestrum of infection. Appropriate intravitreal antibiotic therapy is indicated. If this treatment fails, it may be necessary to search for and remove any visible sequestrum to sterilize the eye. In some cases, total removal of the residual capsule and IOL is necessary.

The possibility of microbial endophthalmitis should be investigated in patients who have persistent uveitis without a previous inflammatory history. (For a more comprehensive discussion of endophthalmitis, see BCSC Section 9, *Intraocular Inflammation and Uveitis.*)

Meisler DM. Intraocular inflammation and extracapsular cataract surgery. *Focal Points: Clinical Modules for Ophthalmologists.* San Francisco: American Academy of Ophthalmology; 1990, module 7.

Capsular Rupture

If capsular rupture occurs during phacoemulsification, nuclear material may enter the posterior segment; the high-fluid-flow state in the anterior chamber exacerbates this risk. The first signs of capsular rupture may be a sudden deepening of the anterior chamber. A radial tear in an anterior curvilinear capsulorrhexis may extend through the capsular fornix into the posterior capsule. A small rupture in the posterior capsule during emulsification of the nucleus can be managed by altering the surgical technique. If the majority of the nucleus remains and the capsular tear is large, further attempts at phacoemulsification should be abandoned. To extract the remaining nuclear fragments mechanically, the surgeon should enlarge the incision and remove the nucleus with a lens loop or spoon in a manner that minimizes vitreous traction or further damage to the capsule.

If only a small portion of the nucleus remains to be aspirated or the rent in the capsule is small, the surgeon, by lowering the infusion bottle, may be able to remove the remaining nuclear material with the phaco tip. Full occlusion of the aspiration port and minimal phacoemulsification power will reduce the risk of further damage to the capsule and aspiration of vitreous. Insertion of a second instrument or lens glide behind the nuclear remnant may help prevent its dislocation into the vitreous. Alternatively, viscoelastic can be introduced posteriorly to the fragment in an effort to float it anteriorly. If the nuclear material drops posteriorly but is still visible, and the surgeon is familiar with pars plana techniques, a posterior assisted levitation maneuver may be attempted. A spatula or viscoelastic cannula is placed through a stab incision in the pars plana and used to elevate the nuclear fragment into the anterior segment. Retrieval of nuclear fragments from the deep vitreous is not recommended.

If the nuclear fragment is not visible, or if the surgeon is not experienced with pars plana incisions, an anterior vitrectomy should be performed with an aspirating guillotine cutter, and the peripheral cortical material should be removed. A 2-port anterior vitrectomy, separating infusion from the aspiration/cutting instrument, facilitates the removal of vitreous from the anterior segment of the eye. If the surgeon is familiar with the technique, the aspiration/cutting instrument may be placed through a pars plana incision and directly visualized in the posterior segment through the pupil while irrigation is continued through the limbus or cornea. This directs flow posteriorly and reduces the amount of vitreous that migrates into the anterior segment. Alternatively, both the irrigation and aspiration/cutting instruments may be placed through 2 separate limbal or corneal incisions. An IOL of choice may be inserted after confirmation of capsular integrity. The wound should then be sutured closed. If posteriorly dislocated nuclear material remains, it should be approached within 1–2 weeks by a vitreoretinal surgeon using a pars plana vitrectomy technique. Retained lens material, especially nuclear material, is often associated with elevated intraocular pressure, significant inflammation, and corneal edema. Following are some guidelines on managing posteriorly dislocated lens fragments for the anterior segment surgeon:

- Attempt retrieval only if fragments are visible and easily accessible.
- Perform anterior vitrectomy to avoid vitreous prolapse.

- Insert IOL when safe and indicated, preferably by capsular fixation, but into the ciliary sulcus or anterior chamber as necessary.
- Perform standard wound closure and viscoelastic removal.
- Prescribe frequent postoperative topical corticosteroids, NSAIDs and IOP-lowering agents.
- Provide referral for prompt vitreoretinal consultation.

If a small rent appears in the posterior capsule during aspiration of cortex without rupture of the vitreous face, the surgeon should attempt to remove the residual cortex without expanding the tear. With viscoelastic to stabilize the anterior chamber, some surgeons use forceps to convert the tear into a round capsulorrhexis that will not spread equatorially. Residual cortex can then be removed from the peripheral lens capsule using low irrigation and aspiration flow to avoid disruption of the hyaloid face. Some surgeons prefer a manual technique, using a cannula attached to a handheld syringe to remove residual cortex after capsular rupture, thereby avoiding any pressure from irrigation.

If larger posterior capsule tears occur, or when the anterior hyaloid face is broken, a vitrectomy is recommended to facilitate the removal of the residual cortex and the subsequent placement of an IOL. A vitrectomy can also prevent the development of vitreomacular traction from the IOL or the wound. Vitreous loss during cataract surgery is associated with an increased risk of retinal detachment and endophthalmitis.

Fishkind WJ. The torn posterior capsule: prevention, recognition, and management. *Focal Points: Clinical Modules for Ophthalmologists.* San Francisco: American Academy of Ophthalmology; 1999, module 4.

Monshizadeh E, Samiy N, Haimovici R. Management of retained intravitreal lens fragments after cataract surgery. *Surv Ophthalmol.* 1999;43:397–404.

Vilar NF, Flynn HWJr, Smiddy WE, et al. Removal of retained lens fragments after phacoemulsification reverses secondary glaucoma and restores visual acuity. *Ophthalmology.* 1997;104:787–792.

Corneal Melting

Keratolysis, or sterile melting of the cornea, may occur following cataract extraction. It is most frequently associated with preexisting tear-film abnormalities resulting from keratoconjunctivitis sicca, Sjögren syndrome, or collagen vascular diseases such as rheumatoid arthritis. Preoperative recognition of these predisposing factors is valuable because the frequent perioperative use of topical lubricants can lessen morbidity. Punctal plug placement or lateral tarsorrhaphy may also be performed at the time of surgery.

Severe stromal melting has also been reported with postoperative use of topical NSAIDs, in part due to the epithelial toxicity and hypoesthesia induced by these drugs. A generic form of diclofenac was most frequently implicated, presumably due to matrix metalloproteinase expression induced by a solubilizer in the topical formulation.

Persistent epithelial defects accompanied by stromal dissolution require intensive treatment with nonpreserved topical lubricants. Additional treatment modalities to encourage epithelialization and arrest stromal melting include punctal occlusion, bandage contact lenses, tarsorrhaphy, serum eye drops (containing epithelial growth factor), and systemic tetracyclines. The prophylactic use of topical antibiotics must be monitored closely. After a week's application, many topical antibiotics begin to cause secondary toxic effects that may inhibit epithelial healing. Treatment of any underlying collagen vascular disease with systemic immunosuppressive therapy such as methotrexate, cyclophospha-mide, and cyclosporine may be necessary.

If the disease continues to progress in spite of medical therapy, the surgeon may undertake amniotic membrane transplantation or lamellar or penetrating keratoplasty. Because corneal melting may recur even with grafted tissue, the physician must maintain intensive lubrication and consider management of any underlying systemic diseases in these cases.

Wound Leak or Filtering Bleb

Filtration of aqueous fluid through the wound may be noted postoperatively. The filtra-tion tends to be self-limited and may respond to observation accompanied by patching and the use of topical and systemic drugs to reduce aqueous production. Reducing or discontinuing postoperative corticosteroids is a way to encourage inflammation and more prompt wound healing.

If filtration persists, a bleb may develop. In the absence of symptoms, observation only is indicated. In the presence of irritation, tearing, contact lens intolerance, infection, a shallow anterior chamber, or significant hypotony, the physician may consider inter-vention. Techniques vary considerably and consist of procedures to enhance inflamma-tion in the wound and thus seal the leak by cicatrization of the bleb. Techniques include the use of light cautery, penetrating diathermy, and cryotherapy, as well as the application of cyanoacrylate glue and the application of dilute solutions of trichloroacetic acid directly to the bleb. Alternatively, the surgeon may consider revising the wound in the early phase when wound healing is not yet complete. In chronic cases, simple suturing may not be sufficient, and a lamellar or patch keratoplasty may be necessary.

Iridodialysis

Iridodialysis, the tearing of the iris at its root or insertion, may occur intraoperatively as a result of the manipulation of intraocular tissues. Insertion of the phaco tip or IOL can sometimes damage the iris. If the iridodialysis is optically and cosmetically insignificant, it can be left alone. More extensive iridodialysis that could cause optical or cosmetic problems may require surgical attachment of the iris root to the wound with permanent monofilament suture.

Cyclodialysis

Cyclodialysis, the separation of the ciliary body from its insertion at the scleral spur, also may occur as a result of surgical manipulation of intraocular tissue. Gonioscopic obser-vation shows a deep angle recess with a gap between the sclera and the ciliary body.

Repair of a cyclodialysis cleft is often indicated to relieve prolonged hypotony; closure can be achieved by applying argon laser photocoagulation to the cleft or by suturing the ciliary body back into place.

Ciliary Block Glaucoma

Ciliary block glaucoma, also known as *malignant glaucoma* or *aqueous misdirection,* results from the posterior misdirection of aqueous into the vitreous body. This misdirection displaces the lens–iris diaphragm anteriorly, causing the central and peripheral portions of the anterior chamber to become very shallow, and leads to a secondary elevation of IOP as a consequence of angle obstruction. This condition occurs most commonly after intraocular surgery in eyes with prior angle-closure glaucoma, but it can also occur in eyes with open angles after cataract surgery or various laser procedures. Ciliary block glaucoma is characterized by a shallow anterior chamber and elevated IOP. It must be differentiated from pupillary block, suprachoroidal hemorrhage, and choroidal detachment.

This posterior diversion of aqueous into the vitreous body after ocular surgery can elevate the IOP despite the presence of a patent iridectomy or iridotomy. Thus, ciliary block glaucoma is not relieved by simple iridectomy but requires either intense medical therapy or surgical therapy. *Medical treatment* consists of intensive cycloplegia/mydriasis with agents such as atropine 1% and phenylephrine 10% 4 times a day to attempt to move the lens–iris diaphragm posteriorly. This therapy is coupled with aqueous suppressants (such as beta blockers, alpha agonists, and oral carbonic anhydrase inhibitors) and hyperosmotic agents (such as oral glycerine, isosorbide, or intravenous mannitol) to reduce aqueous production and lower the IOP. Miotics should be avoided because they make ciliary block glaucoma worse by exacerbating the anterior displacement of the lens–iris diaphragm. Medical therapy is successful in 50% of these cases. Surgical intervention consists of maneuvers to disrupt the anterior hyaloid face and vitreous in order to reestablish a channel for aqueous to come forward. Techniques include mechanical disruption with a knife, use of the Nd:YAG laser, or pars plana vitrectomy. (See also BCSC Section 10, *Glaucoma.*)

> Lundy DM. Ciliary block glaucoma. *Focal Points: Clinical Modules for Ophthalmologists.* San Francisco: American Academy of Ophthalmology. 1999, module 3.

Retained Lens Material

During lens removal, lens fragments may remain in the anterior chamber angle or in the posterior chamber behind the iris, or they may migrate into the vitreous cavity if zonular dehiscence or posterior capsular rupture occurs. This complication is thought to occur more commonly with phacoemulsification than with ECCE, and some experts believe the incidence is about 0.3%. (See Capsular Rupture earlier in this chapter for a discussion of the surgical handling of this intraoperative complication.)

Patients with retained lens fragments present with varying degrees of inflammation, depending on the size of the lens fragment, the type of lens material, amount of time elapsed since surgery, and the patient's individual response. The clinical signs of retained lens material may include uveitis, glaucoma, corneal edema, and vitreous opacities causing profound visual loss.

Retained lens material does not necessarily require surgical intervention. In general, cortical material is better tolerated and more likely to resorb over time than is nuclear material, which persists longer and is more likely to incite a significant inflammatory reaction and elevated IOP, even in small amounts. In addition, smaller fragments of lens material are better tolerated than larger pieces, for the same reasons.

Observation is warranted for patients with small amounts of retained lens material in the hope that the lens material will be resorbed. Inflammation should be controlled with corticosteroid and nonsteroidal anti-inflammatory drops and cycloplegics. IOP can be controlled with topical agents and systemic carbonic anhydrase inhibitors. Surgical intervention may be necessary to remove residual lens material in the following situations:

- presence of a very large and visually significant amount of lens material
- increased inflammation not readily controlled with topical medications
- medically unresponsive elevated IOP resulting from the inflammation
- associated retinal detachment or retinal tears
- associated endophthalmitis

If the posterior capsule is intact, simple aspiration of residual cortex through an anterior incision may be carried out using an irrigation/aspiration instrument. If there is a defect in the posterior capsule, pars plana vitrectomy and removal of lens material are more appropriate. When such major intervention is necessary, retained lens material should be removed from the vitreous by a surgeon skilled in pars plana vitrectomy techniques. Recent studies have reported that the vitreoretinal surgeon can delay intervention up to 7–14 days following the initial cataract surgery without jeopardizing the successful outcome. Chronic glaucoma and CME may be more likely when intervention is delayed more than 3 weeks after the cataract surgery.

Monshizadeh E, Samiy N, Haimovici R. Management of retained intravitreal lens fragments after cataract surgery. *Surv Ophthalmol.* 1999;43:397–404.

Vilar NF, Flynn HW Jr, Smiddy WE, et al. Removal of retained lens fragments after phacoemulsification reverses secondary glaucoma and restores visual acuity. *Ophthalmology.* 1997;104:787–792.

Vitreous Disruption or Incarceration in Wound

Migration of the vitreous through the pupil as a result of rupture of the anterior hyaloid face during surgery can occur as a complication of cataract extraction by any technique. Vitreous traction can lead to retinal breaks and subsequent detachment. Appropriate intraoperative management involves cutting vitreous strands into short segments for removal by a suction cutter or cellulose sponges. The presence of vitreous may be detected by touching or manipulating the wound or iris with a cellulose sponge or spatula. Adherent vitreous will become apparent or will cause movement of the pupil. All vitreous anterior to the posterior capsule should be removed at the time of surgery.

Vitreous in the anterior chamber may lead to chronic ocular inflammation with or without associated CME. The pupil may also be distorted, exposing the edge of the IOL with resultant glare. If there is significant glare from a distorted pupil, or if symptomatic uveitis or CME is unresponsive to topical anti-inflammatory therapy, it may be appropriate to consider disruption of vitreous incarcerated in the wound by means of Nd:YAG laser or vitrectomy techniques. A vitrectomy should be performed if the vitreous extends through the wound to the ocular surface because the vitreous may act like a wick, enabling bacteria to gain entrance into the eye and increasing the risk of endophthalmitis (vitreous wick syndrome). In cases showing considerable corneal compromise, a posterior, rather than an anterior, vitrectomy approach may be preferable to reduce the inevitable surgical trauma to the cornea.

Induced Astigmatism

Postoperative astigmatism may be caused by tight radial sutures, which steepen corneal curvature in the axis of the suture. Following ECCE through a superior incision, up to 2 D of with-the-rule astigmatism will usually diminish with time and may make suture removal unnecessary. Removing one or more sutures 6–8 weeks postoperatively can reduce excessive astigmatism. If more than one suture is to be removed, it may be preferable to remove adjacent sutures in a series of visits rather than all at once. Removal of too many sutures too early in the postoperative course may result in significant corneal flattening in the axis of the incision or a wound leak, with an attendant increased risk of secondary intraocular infection as a result of the entry of surface organisms into the eye through a suture track. Postoperative astigmatism may also be induced by corneal burns from the phaco tip; suture removal 6–8 weeks after surgery generally reduces astigmatism in this setting.

For further discussion of wound construction and astigmatism, see Chapter 8.

Pupillary Capture

Postoperative pupillary capture can occur for a variety of reasons, including formation of synechiae between the iris and underlying posterior capsule, improper placement of the IOL haptics, shallowing of the anterior chamber, or anterior displacement of the posterior chamber IOL optic. The latter is associated with placement of nonangulated IOLs in the ciliary sulcus, upside-down placement of an angulated IOL so that it angles anteriorly, or positive vitreous pressure behind the lens optic. Placement of a posteriorly angulated posterior chamber IOL in the capsular bag decreases the likelihood of pupillary capture.

Usually, pupillary capture is purely a cosmetic issue: the patient is otherwise asymptomatic and can be left untreated. Occasionally, pupillary capture can cause problems with glare, photophobia, chronic uveitis, and even monocular diplopia. Pharmacologic manipulation of the pupil with mydriatics to attempt to free the iris is sometimes successful. If conservative management fails, surgical intervention may be required to free the iris, break the synechiae, or reposition the lens (Figs 9-4, 9-5).

Epithelial Downgrowth

Epithelial downgrowth is a rare complication of intraocular surgery that occurs even less frequently with today's cataract surgery techniques. The condition is characterized by a sheet of epithelium growing down from the surgical wound and covering the corneal endothelium and/or iris surfaces. One possible explanation for this condition is that epithelial cells are introduced into the anterior chamber during surgery, and they adhere to intraocular structures and begin to proliferate as a cellular membrane. Another theory is that a sheet of epithelium from the ocular surface grows into the wound (possibly because the wound is not watertight), and this cellular membrane proliferates onto the posterior corneal and iris surfaces.

The clinical signs of epithelial downgrowth include elevated IOP, clumps of cells floating in the anterior chamber, a visible retrocorneal membrane (usually with overlying corneal edema), an abnormal iris surface, and pupillary distortion. The mechanism for elevated IOP is outflow obstruction caused by the growth of the epithelial membrane over the trabecular meshwork or by epithelial cells clogging the meshwork. Diagnosis of epithelial downgrowth is confirmed with the argon laser; argon laser burns applied to the membrane or the iris surface will appear white if epithelial cells are present. Many complex surgical procedures have been suggested for treating this condition, including local application of 5-fluorouracil, but none have been uniformly successful. In some patients, palliative surgery with glaucoma valve implants for IOP control and comfort is indicated.

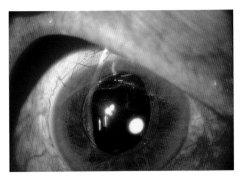

Figure 9-4 Pupillary capture. *(Photograph courtesy of Karla J. Johns, MD.)*

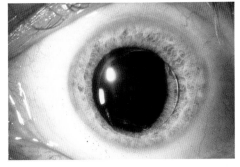

Figure 9-5 Pupillary capture by angled posterior chamber IOL in patient mugged 2 months postoperatively. *(Photograph courtesy of Steven I. Rosenfeld, MD.)*

Capsular Opacification and Contraction

Posterior Capsule Opacification

Overall, the most common complication of cataract surgery by means of ECCE or pha-coemulsification is opacification of the intact posterior capsule. In addition, the introduction of continuous curvilinear capsulorrhexis has been accompanied in some cases by anterior capsule contraction and fibrosis (see the following subsection). Fortunately, posterior capsule opacification is amenable to treatment by means of Nd:YAG posterior capsulotomy.

Capsular opacification stems from the continued viability of lens epithelial cells remaining after removal of the nucleus and cortex. These cells proliferate in several patterns. Where the edges of the anterior capsule adhere to the posterior capsule, a closed space will be reestablished consisting of nucleated bladder cells *(Wedl cells)*, resulting in a *Soemmerring's ring*. If the epithelial cells migrate outward, *Elschnig pearls*, which resemble fish eggs, are formed on the posterior capsule. These pearls can fill the pupil or remain hidden behind the iris. Histopathology shows that each "fish egg" is a nucleated bladder cell, identical to those proliferating within the capsule of a Soemmerring's ring but lying outside the capsule and usually lacking a basement membrane. If the epithelial cells migrate across the anterior or posterior capsule, they may cause capsular wrinkling and opacification. Significantly, the lens epithelial cells are capable of undergoing metaplasia with conversion to myofibroblasts. A matrix of fibrous and basement membrane collagen can be produced by these cells, and contraction of this collagen matrix will cause wrinkles in the posterior capsule, with resultant distortion of vision and glare. Meticulous hydrodissection and attention to complete cortical cleanup are important preventive measures for reducing the likelihood of these events.

Apple DJ, Auffarth GU, Peng A, et al. *Foldable Intraocular Lenses: Evolution, Clinicopathologic Correlations, and Complications.* Thorofare, NJ: Slack; 2000.

Apple DJ, Solomon KD, Tetz MR, et al. Posterior capsule opacification. *Surv Ophthalmol.* 1992;37:73–116.

Caporossi A, Casprini F, Tosi GM, et al. Histology of anterior capsule fibrosis following pha-coemulsification. *J Cataract Refract Surg.* 1998;24:1343–1346.

The reported incidence of posterior capsule opacification varies widely. Factors known to influence this rate include the age of the patient, history of intraocular inflammation, presence of exfoliation syndrome, size of the capsulorrhexis, quality of cortical cleanup, capsular fixation of the implant, lens implant design (particularly a square-edge optic design), lens surface modification, and time elapsed since surgery. In addition, the presence of intraocular silicone oil may dramatically speed the progression of opacity. Anterior capsule opacity appears to be influenced by these same circumstances but is also more likely to occur in cases of a small capsulorrhexis or in the presence of weakened zonules.

Analysis of pooled multiple reports has found the visually significant posterior capsule opacification rate overall to be about 28% at 5 years. Quantitatively measured opacification incidence at 3 years has been reported at 56% for PMMA, 40% for silicone, and 10% for acrylic material, although the Nd:YAG rate is lower. In a large postmortem review, the prevalence of Nd:YAG capsulotomy was 0.9% for acrylic IOLs, 12%–21% for various silicone IOLs, and 27%–33% for PMMA IOLs. Newer generations of silicone materials appear to have a lower rate of opacification. It is now believed that this variation may be due to lens design or anterior capsule overlap rather than lens material.

Apple DJ, Peng Q, Visessook N, et al. Eradication of posterior capsule opacification: documentation of a marked decrease in Nd:YAG laser posterior capsulotomy rates noted in an analysis of 5416 pseudophakic human eyes obtained postmortem. *Ophthalmology.* 2001;108:505–518.

Daynes T, Spencer TS, Doan K, et al. Three-year clinical comparison of 3-piece AcrySof and SI-40 silicone intraocular lenses. *J Cataract Refract Surg.* 2002;28:1124–1129.

Hollick EJ, Spalton DJ, Ursell PG, et al. The effect of polymethylmethacrylate, silicone, and polyacrylic intraocular lenses on posterior capsular opacification 3 years after cataract surgery. *Ophthalmology.* 1999;106:49–55.

Nishi O. Posterior capsule opacification. Part 1: Experimental investigations. *J Cataract Refract Surg.* 1999;25:106–117.

Olsen GM, Olson RJ. Prospective study of cataract surgery, capsulotomy, and retinal detachment. *J Cataract Refract Surg.* 1995;21:136–139.

Schaumberg DA, Dana MR, Christen WG, et al. A systematic overview of the incidence of posterior capsule opacification. *Ophthalmology.* 1998;105:1213–1221.

Anterior Capsule Fibrosis and Phimosis

Capsular fibrosis is associated with clouding of the anterior capsule. If a substantial portion of the IOL optic is covered by the anterior capsule, including portions exposed through the undilated pupil, the patient may become symptomatic when fibrosis occurs. Symptoms may include glare, especially at night owing to natural mydriasis in darkness, or the sensation of a peripheral cloud or haze.

Capsular phimosis is a term used to describe the postoperative contraction of the anterior capsular opening as a result of fibrosis, such that the rim of capsular tissue is also visible through the undilated pupil. Phimosis produces symptoms similar to, and often more pronounced than, fibrosis itself and may cause decentration of an IOL optic. Phimosis occurs more frequently with smaller capsulorrhexis openings, in patients with underlying exfoliation syndrome of the lens, in other disorders with abnormal or asymmetric zonular support (for example, penetrating or blunt trauma, Marfan syndrome, or surgical trauma), and plate haptic posterior chamber IOLs.

Treatment, which should be reserved for symptomatic patients, usually consists of an Nd:YAG laser anterior capsulotomy to enlarge the anterior capsular opening. This procedure is performed in a fashion similar to an Nd:YAG laser posterior capsulotomy, with care taken not to defocus too far posteriorly and damage the underlying IOL with laser pitting. In general, the anterior capsule tissue is tougher and requires more laser power than the posterior capsule.

Nd:YAG Capsulotomy

Use of the Nd:YAG laser is now a standard procedure for treating secondary opacification of the posterior capsule or anterior capsule contraction, although a discission knife can be used through an ab externo corneal incision to open an opacified capsule in special cases.

Indications

The following are indications for Nd:YAG capsulotomy:

- best-corrected visual acuity symptomatically decreased as a result of a hazy posterior capsule
- a hazy posterior capsule preventing the clear view of the ocular fundus required for diagnostic or therapeutic purposes
- monocular diplopia or glare caused by posterior capsule wrinkling or by encroachment of a partially opened posterior capsule into the visual axis of a patient with otherwise clear media and good acuity
- contraction of anterior capsulotomy margins *(capsular phimosis)* encroaching on the visual axis or altering the lens optic position, requiring relaxing incisions

Contraindications

The following are contraindications to Nd:YAG capsulotomy:

- inadequate visualization of the posterior capsule
- an uncooperative patient who is unable to remain still or hold fixation during the procedure (use of a contact lens or retrobulbar anesthesia may enhance the feasibility of a capsulotomy in some of these patients)

Procedure

Nd:YAG laser discission is usually painless and is performed as an outpatient procedure. The surgeon should first adjust the oculars of the microscope-laser delivery system so that the focal point of the helium-neon aiming beam is clearly brought into focus. The pulse energy threshold for puncture of the posterior capsule is generally 0.8–2.0 mJ with either Q-switched or mode-locked systems. To puncture the posterior capsule, the surgeon should use the lowest effective energy output setting. Higher energy levels may be required for areas of dense fibrosis. The Nd:YAG laser emits radiation at a wavelength of 1064 nm and can be operated either in a continuous wave or in the following pulsed modes:

- long-pulsed, 0.1–1.0 ms
- Q-switched, 5–30 ns
- mode-locked, 30–200 ps

The Q-switched and mode-locked systems are the most commonly used in commercially available Nd:YAG lasers.

Observation of the posterior capsule through an undilated pupil can help the surgeon pinpoint the location of the visual axis. The center of the visual axis is the desired site of the opening, which is usually adequate at 3–4 mm in diameter. In some circumstances, larger diameter openings may be required for more complete visualization of the fundus. Dilation is not always necessary for the procedure, but it may be helpful in producing a larger opening in the posterior capsule. Specific landmarks in the posterior capsule near the visual axis should be noted *before* dilation, because the dilated pupil will no longer reveal the visual axis.

A high-plus-power anterior segment laser lens, used with topical anesthesia, improves ocular stability and enlarges the cone angle of the beam, producing an even smaller focus. The smaller-focus diameter facilitates the laser pulse puncture of the capsule, and structures in front of and behind the point of focus are less likely to be damaged (Fig 9-6). If light reflections from the slit-lamp illumination or the aiming beam obscure the area to be treated, the position of the biomicroscope may be adjusted, or the patient can shift fixation slightly.

The increasing preference of surgeons for foldable lens materials has implications for the technique of Nd:YAG capsulotomy. Occasional reports of dislocation of these lenses into the vitreous following capsulotomy have been of concern, particularly with silicone plate haptic lenses. Constructing the capsulotomy in a spiraling circular pattern, rather than in a cruciate pattern, creates an opening less likely to extend radially (Fig 9-7).

If the energy output applied is minimal, the anterior hyaloid face may remain intact. A ruptured anterior hyaloid face will often be kept in check by the presence of a posterior chamber IOL, although vitreous strands occasionally migrate around the lens through

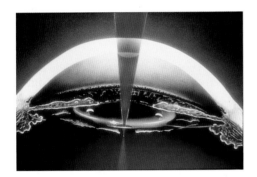

Figure 9-6 Enlarged cone angle of laser beam produces a smaller focus, facilitating laser pulse puncture of the capsule. *(Photograph courtesy of Woodford S. Van Meter, MD.)*

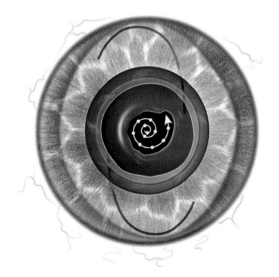

Figure 9-7 Making the series of laser punctures in a spiraling, rather than cruciate, pattern decreases the risk of radial tears. *(Illustration by Christine Gralapp.)*

the pupil. In the event that vitreous moves forward after Nd:YAG laser discission, patients without an iridectomy may develop pupillary block. Although the incidence of pupillary block is very low, patients without a patent iridectomy should be advised to contact their treating physician if pain or other symptoms of pupillary block glaucoma develop after surgery.

Any posterior chamber IOL can be damaged by laser capsulotomy, but the threshold for lens damage appears to be lower for silicone than for other materials. The laser pulse should be focused just behind the posterior capsule, but pulses too far behind the IOL will be ineffective. The safest approach is to focus the laser beam slightly behind the posterior surface of the capsule for initial application, moving subsequent applications anteriorly until the desired puncture is achieved. The surgeon should also search for sites where the capsule might have dropped more posterior to the IOL, because these sites can be treated more safely.

Newland TJ, McDermott ML, Eliott D, et al. Experimental neodymium:YAG laser damage to acrylic, poly(methyl methacrylate), and silicone intraocular lens material. *J Cataract Refract Surg.* 1999;25:72–76.

In cases of anterior capsular contraction, multiple relaxing incisions of the fibrotic ring are applied to relieve the contracting force and create a larger optical opening. Cycloplegic and anti-inflammatory drugs are not routinely necessary. Preoperative and postoperative application of topical apraclonidine hydrochloride (Iopidine) or brimonidine tartrate (Alphagan) is recommended to prevent postoperative IOP elevation.

The success rate of Nd:YAG laser discission for opening the capsule appears to exceed 95%. Occasionally, opacification that is exceptionally thick and dense is not affected by the Nd:YAG laser; these patients may require an invasive surgical procedure using a discission knife or scissors.

Complications

Transient elevation of IOP can appear in a significant number of patients. It is appropriate to treat this prophylactically with a topical alpha-adrenergic agent, and in some patients to monitor postdiscission IOP. Pressure levels peak within 2–3 hours. This elevation appears to be a consequence of obstruction of the outflow pathways by debris or macromolecules scattered by the laser treatment. Elevations respond quickly to topical glaucoma medications, which can be continued for 3–5 days following the procedure. Special precautions should be taken to treat and follow patients with preexisting glaucoma.

Nd:YAG capsulotomy increases the risk of retinal detachment. Approximately half of the retinal detachments following cataract extraction occur within 1 year of surgery, often associated with a posterior vitreous detachment. In many cases, it is difficult to ascertain whether the retinal detachment is related to the capsulotomy or to the cataract surgery itself. High myopia, vitreous trauma, a family history of retinal detachment, and preexisting pathology are risk factors that increase the risk of retinal detachment following Nd:YAG capsulotomy.

CME can occur following Nd:YAG capsulotomy. In patients with a history of previous CME, or in high-risk patients such as those with diabetic retinopathy, the use of topical steroids and nonsteroidal anti-inflammatory agents (pre- and posttreatment) may be beneficial. The risk for retinal detachment and CME may be greater when Nd:YAG capsulotomy is performed within 6 months after cataract surgery.

Javitt JC, Tielsch JM, Canner JK, et al. National outcomes of cataract extraction. Increased risk of retinal complications associated with Nd:YAG laser capsulotomy. The Cataract Patient Outcomes Research Team. *Ophthalmology*. 1992;99:1487–1498.

It is possible for an implant to dislocate into the vitreous cavity following capsulotomy. This complication is more likely to occur with plate haptic silicone implants (especially those with smaller fenestrations) than with any other type of IOL. Nd:YAG capsulotomy should be delayed for 3 months when a plate haptic silicone lens is present to increase the likelihood of capsular fixation.

The future offers increasing opportunity for further reduction of posterior capsule opacification through improved surgical technique, modifications of lens design and materials, and perhaps pharmacologic intervention. Though the incidence of complications with modern Nd:YAG capsulotomy is small, a zero percent opacification rate is the ultimate surgical goal.

Complications of IOL Implantation

Decentration and Dislocation

An IOL may become decentered in the following situations:

- asymmetric haptic placement, with one haptic in the bag and the other in the sulcus
- insufficient zonular or capsular support
- the presence of irregular fibrosis of the posterior capsule

Decentration can produce unwanted glare and reflections or multiple images if the edge of the lens is within the pupillary space. An IOL that is designed for intracapsular fixation is prone to decentration or dislocation when one or both haptics are placed in the sulcus. If zonular support is inadequate, the surgeon should attempt to rotate the IOL to a position where clinical evidence shows sufficient capsule and zonular fibers to support the implant. The use of a trans-iris IOL fixation suture (McCannel suture) may also be considered (Fig 9-8).

Irregular posterior capsule fibrosis gradually distorts and decenters the IOL. Deformation of the implant may render simple rotation insufficient to properly center the IOL. It may become necessary in these cases to reposition the IOL haptics into the ciliary sulcus or replace the capsule–fixated IOL with a posterior chamber sulcus–fixated IOL. If dislocation of the IOL is complete, the surgeon can sublux the optic of the implant into the pupil by means of vitrectomy techniques and use transcorneal iris-fixation sutures to fix the two haptics of the implant. Alternatively, the implant may be removed altogether and replaced with either an anterior chamber IOL or a transsclerally sutured posterior chamber IOL. Subluxation of scleral-fixated sutured IOLs has been reported 3–9 years after implantation with 10-0 polypropylene fixation sutures. Double-fixation

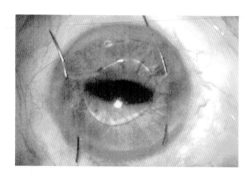

Figure 9-8 McCannel suture. The lens optic is replaced posterior to the iris after retrieving and tying the suture ends through a paracentesis.

techniques and thicker 9-0 polypropylene sutures are currently recommended for scleral fixation of IOLs.

Assia EI, Nemet A, Sachs D. Bilateral spontaneous subluxation of scleral-fixated intraocular lenses. *J Cataract Refract Surg.* 2002;28:2214–2216.

Uveitis-Glaucoma-Hyphema (UGH) Syndrome

The syndrome of uveitis, glaucoma, and hyphema was first described in the context of rigid anterior chamber and closed-loop IOLs. The classic triad or individual elements may occur as a result of inappropriate IOL sizing, contact between the implant and vascular structures, or defects in implant manufacturing. It can also appear as an apparently idiosyncratic reaction of the patient to the implant. Uveitis, glaucoma, and/or hyphema may respond to treatment with topical anti-inflammatory medications or antiglaucoma medications. If the symptoms are not alleviated sufficiently by medical therapy, or if inflammation threatens either retinal or corneal function, IOL removal must be considered. This procedure may be very complicated because of inflammatory scars, particularly in the angle. If such scarring is present, the surgeon must tease the implant out from the synechial tunnels. It may be necessary to amputate the haptics from the optic and remove the lens piecemeal to minimize trauma to the eye or to leave portions of the haptics in place. Early lens explantation may reduce the risk of corneal decompensation and CME.

Corneal Edema and Pseudophakic Bullous Keratopathy

Patients with underlying corneal endothelial dysfunction such as Fuchs corneal dystrophy are at risk for developing postoperative corneal edema, even after smooth, nontraumatic surgery. Corneal edema may occur secondary to surgical trauma or to toxic substances inadvertently introduced into the anterior chamber, or it may be associated with a particular type of IOL, such as an iris-fixated or closed-loop flexible anterior chamber IOL. Vitreous contact with the corneal endothelium and glaucoma may further complicate this condition. Significant chronic corneal edema results in bullous keratopathy, which is associated with reduced visual acuity, irritation, foreign-body sensation, epiphora, and occasional infectious keratitis (Fig 9-9).

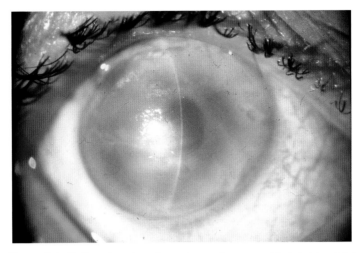

Figure 9-9 Bullous keratopathy. *(Photograph courtesy of Karla J. Johns, MD.)*

In its early stages, corneal edema after cataract surgery can be controlled by the use of topical hyperosmotic agents, topical corticosteroids, and, occasionally, bandage (therapeutic) contact lenses. Over time, subepithelial scarring may develop, resulting in a decrease in bulla formation and discomfort. Decreased visual acuity, recurrent infectious keratitis, and symptoms of pain are possible indications for penetrating keratoplasty. The likelihood of obtaining a clear graft is high, but coexisting CME may limit full recovery of visual acuity. Bulla formation and pain associated with bullous keratopathy may be alleviated with phototherapeutic keratectomy or anterior stromal micropuncture, but it may recur. Cautery of the corneal epithelium and anterior stroma can also reduce formation of bullae but could lead to bacterial keratitis or stromal melting. In the case of an eye with little or no visual potential, a Gundersen conjunctival flap or an amniotic membrane graft is an option that does not carry the greater risks of penetrating keratoplasty. (See also BCSC Section 8, *External Disease and Cornea.*)

Wrong Power IOL

Placement of an incorrect power IOL is usually the result of a preoperative error in axial length measurement or keratometry readings. Choosing the correct power IOL is more difficult in patients undergoing simultaneous penetrating keratoplasty, those with silicone oil in the vitreous cavity, and those who have had prior refractive surgery. Special care should be taken in selecting an IOL in these cases (see Primary Intraocular Lens Implantation in Adults, IOL Power Determination). Inverting the IOL upon insertion so that the angulation of the optic is anterior rather than posterior changes the effective power of the IOL. Manufacturing defects or mislabeling are rarely the cause. Incorrect lens power should be suspected early in the postoperative course when the uncorrected visual acuity is less than expected and is confirmed by refraction. The surgeon should discuss this complication and possible solutions with the patient.

If the magnitude of the implant error is likely to produce symptomatic anisometropia, the surgeon can consider several options: replacing the IOL with one in the appropriate power, inserting a piggyback IOL, or performing a secondary keratorefractive procedure.

IOL Design, Glare, and Opacification

In addition to lens decentration and capsular opacification, glare can result when the diameter of the IOL optic is smaller than the scotopic pupil. Optics with a square-edge design may also be more prone to producing glare. A number of IOLs have developed intralenticular opacities after implantation. "Glistenings" visible in some early acrylic lenses were occasionally visually significant. Calcium deposition on the surface of hydrophilic acrylic lenses has produced significant visual symptoms, leading to lens explantation.

Werner L, Apple DJ, Escobar-Gomez M, et al. Postoperative deposition of calcium on the surfaces of a hydrogel intraocular lens. *Ophthalmology*. 2000;107:2179–2185.

CHAPTER 10

Cataract Surgery in Special Situations

Cataract in Children

Surgical Planning

The surgical management of cataracts in the pediatric age group requires consideration of a wide range of factors unique to this population. The risk of amblyopia has an impact on the timing of surgery and the method of aphakic correction. The patient's parents play a critical role in the postoperative care of the eye and the treatment of amblyopia. They must understand that a successful visual result depends on more than the surgical procedure; it also depends on their ability to maintain adequate aphakic correction and follow through with amblyopia therapy. The surgeon must be certain that the parents' expectations of a successful visual result are realistic, given the child's age and type of cataract.

The child may have to undergo repeated general anesthesia for surgery and for some postoperative examinations. Optimal management often requires the coordinated efforts of several physicians: the ophthalmologist who will perform the surgery and direct the postoperative amblyopia therapy, the pediatrician, the contact lens specialist, and the anesthesiologist.

Bilateral congenital cataracts

The management of bilateral congenital cataracts depends on the etiology and the degree to which the cataracts interfere with vision. Patients with small axial cataracts often maintain good vision if their pupils are continuously dilated with mydriatic drops. Severe bilateral cataracts must be removed if the patient is to develop functional vision. Current concepts of amblyopia and the normal development of the fixation reflex necessitate timely cataract removal when the visual axis is significantly obstructed. Children with profound bilateral amblyopia from cataracts develop nystagmus at approximately 3 months of age because the fixation reflex normally develops by that time. Once nystagmus has developed, it is likely to persist even if the cataracts are subsequently removed. Visual acuity in eyes with nystagmus and infantile cataracts is rarely better than 20/200 after cataract surgery. The only way to obtain a better visual result is to perform the surgery as early as possible and provide appropriate aphakic correction. Thus, in bilateral, severe cataracts, surgery is recommended on the first eye as soon as possible after diagnosis—

ideally, prior to 3 months of age. If all goes well with the first eye, removal of the cataract from the fellow eye should follow promptly. It has been suggested that surgeries be separated by 2 weeks for children under the age of 2 years and by 1 month for children over the age of 2 years.

Peterseim MW, Wilson ME. Bilateral intraocular lens implantation in the pediatric population. *Ophthalmology.* 2000;107:1261–1266.

Unilateral congenital cataract

With a unilateral congenital or infantile cataract, the prognosis for useful vision in the affected eye depends on prompt restoration of a clear visual axis, correction of aphakia, and aggressive treatment of amblyopia. Studies have suggested that intervention before 6 weeks of age may minimize the effects of congenital unilateral deprivation on the visual system and provide for optimal rehabilitation of visual acuity. Although excellent results have been reported with optimal care in such children, the overall prognosis is guarded, regardless of the technique used for refractive correction and amblyopia therapy. Before agreeing to early surgery, parents must understand the hardships that aphakic correction and occlusion therapy will cause during the first decade of the child's life and realize that, despite sometimes heroic efforts, the overall visual results may be disappointing.

Birch EE, Stager DR. The critical period for surgical treatment of dense congenital unilateral cataract. *Invest Ophthalmol Vis Sci.* 1996;37:1532–1538.

Surgical Technique

Cataract surgery in children is similar in many respects to that in adults, although significant differences exist. Features unique to a child's eye include changing axial length, corneal curvature, and lenticular refracting power; increased tissue reactivity; lower scleral rigidity; more elastic capsule; smaller size; potential for amblyopia; and long life span after cataract removal. Also, compared to adults, children have an enhanced inflammatory and fibrotic response to cataract surgery.

Over the past decade, advances in adult cataract surgery techniques have been transferred to pediatric cataract removal. Although a temporal approach is possible in children, just as in adults, a superior incision beneath a scleral tunnel is thought to provide the child with a more secure wound, at less risk from a subsequent traumatic injury. Scleral tunnel incisions help maintain the anterior chamber during the procedure. Scleral wounds should be closed with suture. Incisions that self-seal in adults require suture in pediatric patients. High-viscosity viscoelastics facilitate the anterior capsulotomy. Due to the increased elasticity of the capsule, the surgeon should aim for a smaller opening due to the predictable expansion of the capsulotomy. Several variations of pediatric anterior capsulorrhexis have been described, including mechanized anterior capsulotomy using a vitrector. If an intraocular lens is to be implanted, it is important to avoid radial tears that ultimately could result in intraocular lens displacement. The anterior capsulotomy should be large enough not to contract and reduce the effective pupil size but not so large that peripheral anterior synechiae form between the iris and edge of the capsule and exposed lens.

Congenital cataracts are removed by simple aspiration or lensectomy. The nucleus and cortex in young children tend to be gummy and do not aspirate in the same manner as the adult lens cortex. Cannulas with a 0.3-mm port, commonly used in adult irrigation/aspiration systems, are less effective in this situation than the larger aspiration port of a vitrectomy instrument or phaco tip.

In cataracts with associated blood vessel anomalies, such as persistent fetal vasculature (PFV, previously known as "persistent hyperplastic primary vitreous"), intraoperative bleeding may occur. Vitrectomy instrumentation is often used in such cases to assist with hemostasis and to remove the posterior lens capsule, abnormal membranes, and anterior vitreous.

In the past, complete or large posterior capsulectomy and limited anterior vitrectomy were recommended because of the high incidence of lens capsule opacification and secondary membrane formation across the intact hyaloid face and capsule remnants, which contribute to sensory deprivation amblyopia. More recent studies have shown that with current surgical techniques and implant lenses, the posterior capsule opacified, on average, 2 years after surgery regardless of age. Consideration should be given to primary posterior capsulotomy and anterior vitrectomy at the time of lens implant in children who are not expected to be candidates for Nd:YAG capsulotomy within 18 months. According to published recommendations, the age for patients undergoing primary posterior capsulotomy ranges from 2 years or younger to 5 or 6 years or younger. Techniques for posterior capsulotomy include posterior capsulorrhexis (with optic capture if an intraocular lens is implanted) and pars plana approach with mechanical capsulotomy and anterior vitrectomy. Both of these techniques prevent posterior capsular opacification and decrease the possibility of secondary membrane formation.

If a secondary opacification occurs, an alternative approach to its treatment is an Nd:YAG laser posterior capsulotomy; however, this procedure is more easily performed in children older than 6 years. If an IOL is present, poor fixation may result in lens pitting. The posterior capsule in children is often thick and may require higher laser energy levels for discission than those used in an adult.

Enyedi LB, Peterseim MW, Freedman SF, et al. Refractive changes after pediatric intraocular lens implantation. *Am J Ophthalmol.* 1998;126:772–781.

Kohnen T. Visual axis opacification after pediatric intraocular lens implantation. *J Cataract Refract Surg.* 2001;27:1141–1142.

Kugelberg M, Zetterstrom C. Pediatric cataract surgery with or without anterior vitrectomy. *J Cataract Refract Surg.* 2002;28:1770–1773.

O'Keefe M, Fenton S, Lanigan B. Visual outcomes and complications of posterior chamber intraocular lens implantation in the first year of life. *J Cataract Refract Surg.* 2001;27:2006–2011.

Pandey SK, Wilson ME, Trivedi RH, et al. Pediatric cataract surgery and intraocular lens implantation: current techniques, complications, and management. *Int Ophthalmol Clin.* 2001;41:175–196.

Plager DA, Lipsky SN, Snyder SK, et al. Capsular management and refractive error in pediatric intraocular lenses. *Ophthalmology.* 1997;104:600–607.

Stager DR Jr, Weakley DR Jr, Hunter JS. Long-term rates of PCO following small incision foldable acrylic intraocular lens implantation in children. *J Pediatr Ophthalmol Strabismus.* 2002;39:73–76.

Tsao K, Kazlas M. The pediatric cataract. In: Pineda R, Espaillat A, Perez VL, et al, eds. *The Complicated Cataract: The Massachusetts Eye and Ear Infirmary Phacoemulsification Practice Handbook.* Thorofare, NJ: Slack; 2001:129–140.

Postoperative Care

Infants and young children require a more aggressive course of topical corticosteroids to reduce the inflammatory reaction to surgery than do adults. Cycloplegia with cyclopentolate 1% or 2%, scopolamine 0.25%, or atropine 1% drops for about 1 month postoperatively is advised.

Complications

Although any of the complications discussed in Chapter 9 can occur in children, glaucoma, retinal detachment, and opacification of retained posterior capsule are the more frequent late complications of congenital cataract surgery. Glaucoma has been reported to occur in 13%–24% of the eyes of children with pediatric cataracts. There have been recent reports, however, of a reduced incidence of glaucoma in children receiving an IOL. Some surgeons advocate that a peripheral iridectomy be performed prophylactically at the time of surgery to prevent later angle-closure glaucoma. Parents should be informed that these children will require follow-up care for their entire lives. There is also a high prevalence of ocular hypertension after pediatric cataract surgery.

Egbert JE, Wright MM, Dahlhauser KF, et al. A prospective study of ocular hypertension and glaucoma after pediatric cataract surgery. *Ophthalmology.* 1995;102:1098–1101.

Prognosis

The visual prognosis for congenital cataract depends on the age of the child at the time of surgery, the severity of the opacity, whether the cataract is unilateral or bilateral, and the degree of compliance with aphakic correction and amblyopia therapy. Visually significant cataracts virtually always result in deprivation amblyopia if left untreated.

Advances in surgical technique and contact lens technology, along with early diagnosis and treatment, have resulted in significant improvements in the prognosis for children with unilateral cataract. Children whose unilateral congenital cataracts are removed within the first 4 months of life may achieve visual acuity of 20/40 or better. When the surgery is performed between 4 and 12 months, visual acuity is reported to be in the range of 20/50 and 20/100. A child up to 5 years old with a unilateral cataract of undetermined age may achieve a visual acuity outcome as good as 20/50, as long as the child has had some normal visual experience prior to the development of the cataract. Associated ocular abnormalities, such as persistent fetal vasculature (PFV) or microphthalmos, often limit the postoperative visual results, even with optimal treatment.

Ruttum MS. Childhood cataracts. *Focal Points: Clinical Modules for Ophthalmologists.* San Francisco: American Academy of Ophthalmology; 1996, module 1.

Correction of Aphakia

Prompt restoration of a focused image is necessary to prevent amblyopia in young children. Retinoscopic refraction is often stable within 1 week after cataract surgery because of the small incision length and rapid wound healing in children. (For a discussion of the treatment of amblyopia, see BCSC Section 6, *Pediatric Ophthalmology and Strabismus.*)

Aphakic spectacles

Children older than 1 year of age (and some younger than 1 year old) with bilateral aphakia may tolerate aphakic spectacles well. Children adapt more easily to the various distortions of spectacles than do adults. Lens size and weight should be minimized to avoid discomfort to the ears and bridge of the nose. Fitting aphakic glasses properly and ensuring compliance in wearing them is usually difficult in children younger than 1 year old. For infants, the lenses of these glasses often require more than 25 D of hyperopic correction. Single-vision near correction may be adequate in very young children, as most of their activities are generally within arm's length. As children grow older, distance correction and near add are more appropriate.

Contact lenses

Contact lens correction is used for monocular or binocular aphakia. It is a well-established method of optical correction for unilateral aphakia in infants. Children can be sedated for lens fittings and examination, and parents can generally be taught to handle insertion and removal for a small child. Soft hydrophilic contact lenses are approved for daily wear and are relatively easy to fit and handle. Silicone soft lenses are approved for extended wear and will be available in a greater range of powers in the future (current range +6.00 to −8.00). Removal on a weekly basis is typical, although the risk of infectious keratitis and other complications increases with overnight lens wear. Rigid gas-permeable lenses are less costly, but they are more complicated to fit and must be removed each day. Visual results in aphakia corrected with a contact lens can be quite good, but a significant physical, emotional, and economic commitment is required from the parents.

Intraocular lens implantation

The advent of improved microsurgical techniques and instrumentation, high-quality posterior chamber lens implants, and viscoelastics has moved IOL implantation in children from a purely investigational procedure to a more mainstream approach. Studies that have compared the use of contact lenses to IOLs for the correction of aphakia in this setting have shown improved binocularity in children with IOLs.

Ocular measurements used to calculate the intraocular lens power in children may need to be done under general anesthesia at the time of surgery. Some surgeons select an IOL power with a refractive goal of emmetropia in patients over 4 years of age; others aim for hyperopia of varying amounts to allow for growth of the eye and resultant refractive power changes.

The use of bilateral lens implantation surgery in children under 1 year of age is still controversial, although it has been successfully reported in infants as young as 12 days.

A procedure called "temporary polypseudophakia" has been described in which piggy-back IOLs are implanted. As the child grows and the eye elongates, resulting in myopia, the more anterior posterior chamber IOL is explanted.

Posterior chamber lenses are the preferred IOLs for children, and fixation in the capsular bag is preferable to fixation in the sulcus. The PMMA optic has the longest track record of biocompatibility within the eye; however, optics made of flexible materials that are popular for use in adult cataract surgery are predominantly being used in the pediatric age group.

Secondary lens implantation can also be used in monoaphakic children who were unable to tolerate contact lenses, provided that there is sufficient visual potential to justify the surgery and enough capsular support to allow for adequate lens stability. Anterior chamber IOLs in children are generally not recommended.

Ruttum MS. Childhood cataracts. *Focal Points: Clinical Modules for Ophthalmologists.* San Francisco: American Academy of Ophthalmology; 1996, module 1.

Wilson ME. Management of aphakia in children. *Focal Points: Clinical Modules for Ophthalmologists.* San Francisco: American Academy of Ophthalmology; 1999, module 1.

Wilson ME, Apple DJ, Bluestein EC, et al. Intraocular lenses for pediatric implantation: biomaterials, designs, and sizing. *J Cataract Refract Surg.* 1994;20:584–591.

Wilson ME, Bluestein EC, Wang XH. Current trends in the use of intraocular lenses in children. *J Cataract Refract Surg.* 1994;20:579–583.

Anticipated Poor Wound Healing

Wound healing is often slower than normal in the following groups of patients: the very elderly, those who are chronically debilitated, individuals who are steroid dependent or receiving antimetabolite therapy, and patients with connective tissue diseases, Marfan syndrome, or diabetes. Early or late wound dehiscence may result. Clinical manifestations can include increased corneal astigmatism, filtering bleb at the scleral wound site, or wound leak and hypotony. These patients are also more prone to wound problems related to minor surgical trauma, and, thus, small-incision cataract surgery is preferred in this situation. When used, sutures should be left in place as long as possible. Steroid therapy should be discontinued as soon as the postoperative inflammation has been controlled.

Psychosocial Considerations

Claustrophobia

All surgical candidates should be questioned preoperatively about their ability to tolerate having their face covered or being confined to a small space. Patients who are claustrophobic often do better with general anesthesia. Hypercarbia, which can occur if exhaled CO_2 accumulates under the surgical drapes, can cause even cooperative patients to suddenly become quite anxious. This situation can be avoided by placing a suction catheter under the drape or by venting the CO_2 by some other means.

Dementia or Other Mental Disabilities

It may be difficult to evaluate the functional deficit caused by cataract in patients with dementia or other mental disability. Questioning the patient's caregiver may provide valuable insight into the patient's functional visual impairment. The surgeon frequently gets the best clinical impression of the significance of the cataract based on retinoscopy, slit-lamp, and fundus examinations. The potential for improvement in visual function and the visual needs of the patient should both be carefully considered preoperatively. In some cases, improvement in visual status increases the patient's mental functioning.

Prior to surgery, the surgeon must determine whether the patient can cooperate if local anesthesia is used. Sedating a patient with a mental disability may cause confusion and increased agitation. If the patient cannot cooperate and is otherwise in good health, general anesthesia should be used. In patients with dementia, regression in mental status following general anesthesia is not uncommon. If the patient seems susceptible to ocular trauma postoperatively, small-incision surgery is preferred.

Inability to Communicate With the Patient

Good communication with the patient is a definite advantage, especially during eye surgery with local anesthesia. Patients with hearing loss should be reminded to wear their hearing aids into the operating room. The surgeon and patient should determine how best to communicate prior to surgery. In cases of profound hearing loss, for example, simple hand signals between the patient and anesthesiologist can be helpful. If the surgeon and patient do not speak the same language, an interpreter or a family member can be brought into the operating room.

Systemic Conditions

Anticoagulation Therapy or Bleeding Disorders

Cataract surgery with IOL implantation in patients receiving chronic anticoagulation therapy is associated with a small additional risk of intraoperative or perioperative bleeding in the eye. Retrobulbar and peribulbar anesthetic injections carry the increased risk of retrobulbar hemorrhage. (See Hemorrhage in Chapter 9.) Contact between the implant and vascular intraocular tissues increases the risk of late postoperative hemorrhage within the eye.

The three most common indications for anticoagulation therapy are atrial fibrillation, prosthetic heart valves, and deep-vein thrombosis (DVT). In deciding how to handle a patient on chronic anticoagulation therapy, the surgeon and primary care physician must weigh the systemic risks of stopping anticoagulation with the localized ocular surgical risks of maintaining the therapy. Although no prospective controlled studies have yet been reported, many retrospective reports have shown that maintenance of anticoagulation is relatively safe in intracapsular cataract extraction (ICCE), extracapsular cataract extraction (ECCE), and clear corneal surgery. The main reported complications include subconjunctival hemorrhages, lid ecchymoses, incisional bleeding, and rare hyphemas. The incidence of retrobulbar or choroidal hemorrhages is rare in this population.

The risks must be weighed against the significant systemic risks of transient ischemic attack (TIA), cerebrovascular accident (CVA), myocardial infarction (MI), recurrent DVT, pulmonary embolus, and failure of coronary or peripheral bypass grafts when the anticoagulation is discontinued.

The anticoagulation effects of warfarin sodium (Coumadin) and heparin are far greater than those of platelet-inhibiting medications such as aspirin, dipyridamole (Persantine), clopidogrel (Plavix), and vitamin E. The decision to discontinue anticoagulation therapy before surgery should be made on an individual basis. Whereas it takes 3–5 days to restore normal coagulation after stopping warfarin, it takes at least 10 days to restore normal platelet function after stopping antiplatelet therapy. Patients should be questioned about the use of all medications, including nonprescription items that could affect their coagulation status.

If the patient requires a retrobulbar or peribulbar injection, or a vascular surgical approach is needed, adjustment of the anticoagulation therapy should be discussed with the patient's primary care physician. Although patients with atrial fibrillation or a single episode of DVT can usually have their anticoagulation medication temporarily discontinued, patients with prosthetic heart valves and recurrent DVT often must maintain their anticoagulation. In these and similar cases, decreasing the warfarin dose and lowering the international normalized ratio (INR) may be sufficient.

Evaluation of the coagulation status prior to surgery should be considered for any patient with a condition that might affect clotting ability—for example, chronic liver disease, bone marrow suppression, malabsorption syndrome, or debilitation. A hematology consult is advised in the presence of these conditions or a known bleeding diathesis. Preoperative transfusion of platelets or fresh frozen plasma may reduce the risk from hemorrhage.

Using topical anesthesia with a clear corneal incision and placing the IOL in the capsular bag is an effective way of minimizing the risk of hemorrhage. Many surgeons who routinely use this approach do not require their patients to discontinue anticoagulation therapy prior to surgery. If the surgeon is not comfortable or experienced with these techniques for cataract surgery, referral of the patient to an appropriately qualified surgeon may be considered.

The reverse Trendelenburg position reduces venous congestion and may lessen the risk of hemorrhage associated with anesthetic injection. Patients can undergo cataract surgery with peribulbar or retrobulbar anesthetic injections, but the surgeon should apprise such patients of the increased risk of periocular hemorrhage, and advise him or her to call immediately if the signs or symptoms of a retrobulbar hemorrhage develop.

Carter K, Miller KM. Phacoemulsification and lens implantation in patients treated with aspirin and warfarin. *J Cataract Refract Surg.* 1998;24:1361–1364.

Kearon C, Hirsh J. Management of anticoagulation before and after elective surgery. *N Engl J Med.* 1997;336:1506–1511.

McMahan LB. Anticoagulants and cataract surgery. *J Cataract Refract Surg.* 1988;14:569–571.

Arthritis

Patients with severe arthritis may be less able to cooperate during surgery because of discomfort, but adjusting the position to optimize patient comfort may create technical difficulties for the surgeon. Often, a compromise position can be found that allows the patient to lie still and also gives the surgeon adequate access to the eye. When such a compromise cannot be reached, general anesthesia should be considered. (Patients with marked kyphosis may be poor candidates for general anesthesia because of associated pulmonary disease.) Adjusting the table for optimal surgical access may compromise respiratory function and may increase periorbital venous congestion. Ankylosing spondylitis with the cervical spine frozen in the face-down position offers a challenge in surgical positioning. It may require that the surgeon operate with the head in a vertical position (Fig 10-1). Medications used to treat arthritis, such as aspirin, NSAIDs, and systemic steroids, may increase the risk of intraoperative and perioperative hemorrhage. Systemic steroids and antimetabolite medications may slow postoperative wound healing.

Chronic Obstructive Pulmonary Disease

Nuclear sclerotic cataracts are commonly seen in older patients, but posterior subcapsular cataracts may occur at a younger age in the steroid-dependent *chronic obstructive pulmonary disease (COPD)* population. Medical evaluation should always be part of the

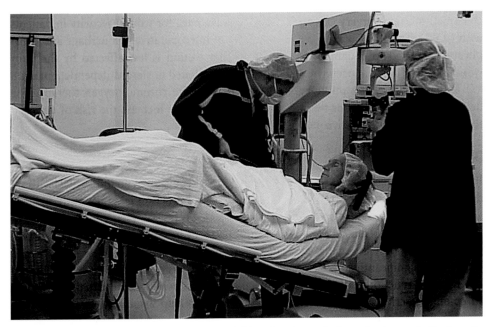

Figure 10-1 Patients with ankylosing spondylitis often have their necks frozen in flexion. To gain surgical access, the operating room bed needs to have flexion capabilities and may need to be tilted. In spite of these maneuvers, the surgeon may be required to operate with the head in a vertical position. A floor-mounted microscope can be maximally tilted to allow adequate visualization.

preoperative planning process, and efforts should be made to assess and maximize pulmonary function before the proposed surgery date. Patients should be encouraged to bring their inhalers into the operating room.

Patients with COPD, bronchitis, or congestive heart failure may have increased venous pressure, which may increase vitreous pressure and make the surgery riskier. Retrobulbar hemorrhage associated with local anesthetic and bleeding during surgery may be more likely. Patients with more severe disease cannot lie flat for the procedure without becoming short of breath. The optimal operating table adjustment for the patient may be awkward for the surgeon. A surgical microscope with forward tilt may be helpful.

Monitored local anesthesia is preferred in these patients. General anesthesia could be considered when the patient cannot endure the required table position but can tolerate this form of anesthesia.

Rosenfeld SI, Litinsky SM, Snyder DA, et al. Effectiveness of monitored anesthesia care in cataract surgery. *Ophthalmology.* 1999;106:1256–1261.

Coughing, both during the procedure and in the immediate postoperative period, is hazardous, particularly with large-incision surgery, and must be accepted as a significant risk in this patient group. Although narcotics can be used judiciously to suppress coughing during surgery, care must be taken to avoid respiratory depression. When there is risk of respiratory depression during surgery, many anesthesiologists prefer to have control of the airway with intubation. Intravenous lidocaine may also be effective as a cough suppressant.

Small-incision surgery can offer a distinct advantage for wound security in patients with COPD. The small wound reduces the risk of intraoperative hemorrhage and complications related to coughing. Further, a smaller wound is less affected by the poor wound healing that can occur in the chronically debilitated or steroid-dependent patient.

Patients with severe pulmonary disease may require chronic oxygen therapy. The delivery system may harbor pathogenic bacteria that may increase the risk of endophthalmitis in the perioperative period.

Diabetes Mellitus

Patients with diabetes develop lens opacities at an earlier age than do individuals without diabetes. Cataract surgery is indicated when the visual function is significantly reduced as a result of the lenticular opacity. It is also indicated if the cataract reduces the view of the retina, thus impeding the diagnosis and treatment of diabetic retinopathy. Cortical cataracts commonly associated with diabetes can greatly reduce the view of the retina before they significantly affect visual function.

Macular function tests, such as the macular photostress test or potential acuity measurements described in Chapter 7, may be needed to help determine visual potential. Fluorescein angiography may help detect the presence of retinopathy and the degree of leakage into the foveal area. If diabetic macular edema is present and the view of the retina is adequate, focal laser treatment should be done preoperatively as nonproliferative diabetic retinopathy can progress following cataract surgery. (See also BCSC Section 12, *Retina and Vitreous.*)

Patients with proliferative retinopathy are more likely to develop neovascularization of the iris and/or worsening of the retinopathy after cataract surgery. Panretinal photocoagulation reduces considerably the risk of iris neovascularization. The risk is greatest for the patient who undergoes ICCE without further treatment. The risk is lower with ECCE with intact posterior capsule. The risk is even lower with small-incision surgery.

Preoperative consultation with the primary care physician regarding local or general anesthesia is recommended in cases of long-standing diabetes because of the increased incidence of associated renal and cardiac disease. In general, if a patient with diabetes is required to fast after midnight on the day of surgery, the oral hypoglycemic agent should be withheld on that day. Insulin-dependent patients should have their insulin dose adjusted after consultation with the primary care provider. Surgery on a patient with diabetes should be done as early in the day as possible. It is essential to have intravenous access to such a patient prior to, during, and immediately after surgery in order to effectively treat a potential hypoglycemic reaction. (For a fuller discussion of ocular surgery in patients with diabetes, see BCSC Section 1, *Update on General Medicine*.)

Extra care should be taken to protect the corneal epithelium during surgery. Corneal abrasions occurring during or after surgery may be slow to heal and can lead to recurrent corneal erosions. Corneal hypoesthesia is not uncommon in a patient with diabetes. Small-incision surgery can minimize any further decrease in corneal sensation. If the pupil is small preoperatively, it may be enlarged during cataract surgery using either multiple sphincterotomies, pupil-stretching techniques, or mechnical iris retractors. A generous anterior capsulotomy and complete cortical cleanup will enhance the view of the retinal periphery.

Patients with diabetes are poor candidates for long-term aphakic contact lens wear, and aphakic spectacles limit visual function. Thus, when possible, a posterior chamber IOL should be inserted. Silicone IOLs can develop condensation during pars plana vitrectomy and thus may be a relative contraindication for individuals who may require this procedure. A larger-diameter optic, 6.0 mm or larger, will facilitate diagnosis and treatment of peripheral retinal pathology following cataract surgery. If posterior capsulotomy becomes necessary, the posterior chamber lens will act as a barrier to the anterior movement of vitreous. Anterior chamber lenses should generally not be used in patients with diabetes who are at risk for iris neovascularization.

Obesity

A patient with severe obesity should be evaluated by the primary care physician prior to cataract surgery. The evaluation may reveal associated diseases such as diabetes, hypertension, or sleep apnea that can affect the intraoperative status of the patient. A large blood pressure cuff should be used and extenders added to the sides of the operating table with elbow pads if the patient does not fit properly on the table. The reverse Trendelenburg position is advantageous because it reduces venous congestion. Positioning the patient's head in the neck-flexed position should be avoided because it can obstruct the airway. Intraoperative continuous positive airway pressure is a useful technique to prevent airway obstruction. If retrobulbar or peribulbar anesthetic is used, avoid injecting an excessive volume, which adds to the pressure on the globe. Ocular massage may be performed prior to surgery to reduce orbital pressure. Small-incision cataract surgery using phacoemulsification has made surgery in the obese, bull-necked patient substantially safer, greatly reducing the risk of vitreous loss.

Ocular Conditions

External Eye Disease

Acne rosacea and/or blepharitis

The hallmarks of blepharitis and meibomianitis are collarettes on the lashes, increased vascularization of the lid margins, and plugging of the meibomian gland orifices with frothy discharge on the lid margin (Fig 10-2). Chronic injection of the bulbar conjunctiva may also occur. Patients with acne rosacea have erythema, telangiectasias, papules, and pustules distributed over the cheeks, chin, forehead, and nose. Inflammation of the eyelid margin is often associated, and patients with such inflammation are at greater risk of endophthalmitis. The patient should undertake a preoperative therapeutic regimen of hot compresses, lid scrubs, and antibiotic ointment applied to the lid margins at bedtime. The condition should be controlled prior to surgery. Systemic tetracyclines help control eyelid disease associated with acne rosacea.

Keratoconjunctivitis sicca

Patients with rheumatoid arthritis and Sjögren syndrome present a special challenge to the cataract surgeon. Despite a lack of symptoms preoperatively, keratolysis (corneal

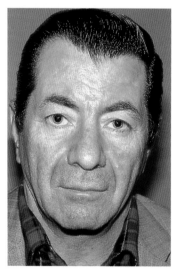 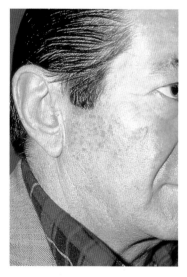

Figure 10-2 Acne rosacea is associated with erythema of the cheeks, nose, chin, and forehead. Papules and pustules are seen in the same distribution. Telangiectatic blood vessels, another common finding, are easily visible in these photographs. *(Photographs courtesy of Mariannette Miller-Meeks, MD.)*

melting) may occur as a result of a combination of denuded corneal epithelium, corneal hypoesthesia related to transection of corneal nerves, and use of topical steroids or non-steroidal anti-inflammatory drops. The dry eye condition should be controlled prior to surgery with liberal use of nonpreserved tears and, if warranted, punctal occlusion. Meticulous care should be taken during the procedure to avoid disturbance or dessication of the corneal epithelium. Small-incision surgery is advantageous.

Close observation in the weeks following surgery is necessary in order to recognize the early signs of trouble. Prolonged use of antibiotics and steroids should be avoided if the wound is stable and postoperative iritis has diminished. Prolonged antibiotic therapy may lead to a toxic keratoconjunctivitis, which may slow postoperative visual rehabilitation. Further, prolonged steroid use can inhibit wound healing and increase the risk of corneal ulceration associated with steroid enhancement of collagenase. Topical NSAIDs have also been associated with a significant risk of corneal melting.

Persistent corneal epithelial defects accompanied by stromal loss may require intensive treatment with topical lubricants, punctal occlusion, bandage contact lens, tarsorrhaphy, and/or amniotic membrane transplant. Active scleritis associated with collagen vascular diseases such as rheumatoid arthritis should be controlled with oral steroid and/or antimetabolite therapy prior to planning cataract surgery to reduce the risk of scleral or corneal necrosis.

Pemphigoid

The inflammation associated with ocular cicatricial pemphigoid should be well controlled with systemic steroid and/or antimetabolite therapy before cataract surgery is considered. Even so, the condition may reactivate several weeks after surgical trauma. Progressive conjunctival scarring induces a severe dry eye condition resulting from loss of meibomian glands and accessory lacrimal glands in the conjunctiva and scarring of the lacrimal gland orifices. These dry eyes are at risk of corneal melting following cataract surgery. Extensive symblepharon or ankyloblepharon may severely limit the surgeon's ability to position the eye and obtain exposure. Traction on the globe induced by the lid speculum may cause vitreous pressure. Corneal scarring may reduce the visibility of anterior segment structures during the procedure. If visualization is adequate, clear corneal surgery is advantageous in patients with pemphigoid. Patients should be warned that even if their disease is controlled preoperatively, any ocular surgery may cause flare-ups.

Corneal Conditions

When evaluating the cataract patient preoperatively, the clinician should determine how much existing corneal pathology contributes to the patient's overall visual reduction. Corneal conditions that disrupt the anterior refractive surface induce irregular astigmatism, which can dramatically reduce visual acuity. The status of the anterior refractive surface can be assessed with keratometry. If the mires are crisp and the astigmatism regular, the corneal surface is intact. The ophthalmologist can determine the contribution of the irregular surface to the patient's diminished visual acuity by placing a suitable hard contact lens (which will mask the irregular astigmatism) on the cornea and performing an overrefraction. Substantial improvement in visual acuity may indicate that the role played by the cataract is relatively minor.

Epithelial basement membrane dystrophy (Fig 10-3) is a commonly encountered corneal condition that, if pronounced in the area of the visual axis, can reduce vision by disrupting the anterior surface. Epithelial debridement may be the preferred procedure in this situation. Stromal opacities in the presence of a pristine anterior refractive surface are less likely to affect visual acuity.

Endothelial dystrophy (Fig 10-4) presents a special challenge to the cataract surgeon, who must predict how well the cornea will survive routine cataract surgery. The best indicator of endothelial function is corneal thickness measured by ultrasonic pachymetry; in general, if the central corneal thickness is less than 640 μm in the early morning (when the cornea is thickest), the corneal status will probably remain stable following routine cataract surgery. A useful clinical indicator of corneal endothelial dysfunction is a history of diurnal visual fluctuations, with vision being worse each morning due to corneal edema. Every effort should be made to minimize trauma to the endothelium in such a case. If the thickness is greater than 640 μm, the cornea is more likely to fail and the patient is better served by a combined procedure of cataract surgery, IOL insertion, and penetrating keratoplasty (PK). This combination is known as a *triple procedure.*

Triple procedure

When a corneal transplant is necessary, and the cataract is visually significant, the cataract is generally removed concomitantly. There are several reasons for also removing a less significant cataract in this situation:

- Cataracts may progress more rapidly after keratoplasty.
- The use of topical steroids after surgery can hasten cataract development.
- Postkeratoplasty cataract surgery may traumatize the grafted endothelium.

The modern triple procedure may be done as an ECCE through an open-sky approach, using a capsulorrhexis with capsular fixation of a posterior chamber lens implant. The capsulorrhexis should be somewhat larger than usual to accommodate nuclear removal and reduce the risk of inadvertent radial tear. Hydrodissection may facilitate separation of the nucleus from the cortex and ease nuclear expression. Cortical removal is easier using a low-flow manual aspiration technique than an automated approach.

Alternatively, if the view through the cornea is adequate, phacoemulsification of the cataract with posterior IOL insertion can be done in the usual fashion followed by penetrating keratoplasty. This procedure has the advantages of reducing the time that the eye is open and having a posterior chamber IOL to stabilize the globe and keep the vitreous in place. After the IOL is inserted, the pupil is constricted and viscoelastic is placed on the exposed optic to protect the graft endothelium. If capsular support is not adequate, a posterior chamber IOL can be sutured to the iris or sclera. Alternatively, a flexible anterior chamber IOL can be used.

The results of the modern triple procedure are excellent. Over 90% of patients will have clear grafts at 1 year, and over 75% will achieve a best-corrected visual acuity of 20/40 or better in the absence of other vision-limiting conditions. Choosing the IOL

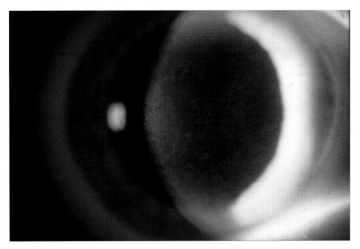

Figure 10-3 Epithelial basement membrane dystrophy. Irregular corneal astigmatism may occur in patients with epithelial basement membrane dystrophy and will appear preoperatively on keratometry as mire irregularity. These patients often have reduced visual acuity related to the abnormal anterior refractive surface. The corneal contribution to decreased acuity may be greater than that from the cataract, in which case the visual improvement after cataract surgery might be less than expected. *(Photograph courtesy of Robert S. Feder, MD.)*

power in this setting can be challenging because the postoperative corneal contour cannot be accurately predicted preoperatively. Most surgeons who perform keratoplasty develop a formula for their specific surgical technique to improve the predictability of the implant power calculation. Patients should be warned of the potential for postoperative anisometropia and the possible need for a contact lens after keratoplasty. Refractive surgery using the excimer laser can reduce symptomatic anisometropia that may occur after all graft sutures have been removed.

Anisometropia can also be corrected with a secondary posterior chamber lens implant. Some corneal surgeons prefer a staged approach to the triple procedure. Performing the corneal transplant first allows for a more accurate IOL power calculation once the cornea has stabilized. This approach increases the stress to the endothelium, delays visual recovery when a visually significant cataract is present at the time of the keratoplasty, and may increase the risk of graft rejection.

Cataract following keratoplasty

Cataract is a well-recognized complication of corneal transplant surgery. It may be a consequence of the same pathology that disrupted the cornea. It may also result from lens trauma during the transplant procedure or from prolonged use of corticosteroids to prevent rejection.

Even though a graft can remain clear with surprisingly low cell counts, it may not survive routine cataract surgery. The surgeon should also look for preoperative corneal thickening and anticipate the possibility that visualization through the graft may be reduced by swelling during the procedure or by instability of the epithelial surface. The

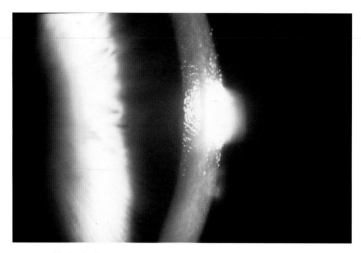

Figure 10-4 Endothelial dystrophy. *(Photograph courtesy of George O. Waring III, MD.)*

risk of graft failure, which is increased when the cornea is subjected to a surgical procedure, can be reduced by minimizing endothelial trauma and controlling postoperative inflammation.

Ideally, cataract surgery should be delayed until the PK sutures are removed so that the corneal contour is stable. If the IOL power is chosen before the corneal contour has stabilized, a change in the refractive power of the cornea can cause significant anisometropia. Posterior chamber lenses are preferred because they minimize the risk of contact between the optic and corneal endothelium. If capsular support is inadequate, a posterior chamber lens can be sutured to the sclera or the iris. However, the additional manipulation needed to secure the lens may have a negative impact on the graft endothelium. Insertion of a flexible open-haptic anterior chamber IOL is another option. The probability of corneal graft survival 5 years after cataract surgery is better than 80%.

Mature cataract/Poor red reflex Capsulorrhexis is more difficult and subject to errant radial tears when a poor red reflex is present, as occurs with a brunescent or mature cataract, or with a vitreous opacity such as a hemorrhage. Corneal opacities that compromise the view of the capsule also make the capsulotomy more challenging. The use of a capsular dye in these situations makes visualization and manipulation of the capsule easier. Two dyes, trypan blue 0.1% and indocyanine green (ICG) 0.5%, currently used for this purpose, appear to be safe for the corneal endothelium. Trypan blue is a more effective capsular stain; it is less expensive and comes as a ready-to-use solution, but it is not available for use in the United States. Indocyanine green has to be reconstituted, but it is available for off-label use. Indocyanine green is prepared by combining 0.5 mL of the diluent supplied by the manufacturer and 4.5 mL of balanced salt solution. The dye is good for 10 hours. At the beginning of surgery, the anterior chamber fluid is exchanged for a single air bubble through a small peripheral paracentesis. A small amount of viscoelastic can then be placed just inside the opening to prevent the air from escaping. Several drops of the ICG are then introduced from the syringe through a 27-gauge cannula onto the surface of the anterior capsule and wiped to distribute across the surface. Viscoelastic is then exchanged for the air and residual dye. The main cataract incision is constructed and the capsulotomy performed. In mature cataracts, the capsule is often more brittle (less elastic) and requires more frequent regrasping of the capsular edge to direct the tear. It has been reported that hydrophilic acrylic lenses with a high water content can be permanently stained and discolored by some ophthalmic dyes.

Pandey SK, Werner L, Wilson ME, Jr, et al. Anterior capsule staining. Techniques, recommendations and guidleline for surgeons. *Indian J Ophthalmol.* 2002;50:157–159.

Werner L, Apple DJ, Crema AS, et al. Permanent blue discoloration of a hydrogel intraocular lens by intraoperative trypan blue. *J Cataract Refract Surg.* 2002;28:1279–1286.

Cataract following refractive surgery

The development of cataract after radial keratotomy (RK) is a rare complication generally associated with perforation of the cornea during surgery. Prolonged use of topical steroids after refractive surgery may also induce cataract. Although most patients undergoing refractive surgery for myopia are young, the later development of cataract in these patients through aging, trauma, medications, or other causes has provided some experience with the risks and complications to be considered when performing cataract surgery.

The most significant problem encountered in RK patients is the instability of the refractive result after cataract surgery. Patients may experience a significant hyperopic shift caused by early postoperative flattening due to corneal edema. Even though the flattening may regress, the resulting corneal curvature cannot be predicted by preoperative keratometry readings. Fluctuating refractive error can occur, along with increased glare, similar to that experienced after the refractive procedure. The surgeon should anticipate visual interference during the cataract procedure, because the RK incisions create reflections from the microscope light. In addition, the multiple deep incisions may also increase the likelihood of anterior chamber shallowing during the procedure. If a corneal incision is used, it must not cross prior RK incisions or the cornea will not be stable.

Intraoperative visualization of the cataract following photorefractive keratectomy (PRK) is a problem only in the setting of anterior stromal haze. The kind of progressive refractive effect seen after RK does not occur in the PRK patient. Superficial haze is not a problem after laser-assisted in situ keratomileusis (LASIK), but extensive epithelial ingrowth and scarring from postoperative infection or an inadvertent buttonhole in the flap could compromise the surgeon's view of the cataract. If a corneal incision is used, damage to the LASIK flap should be avoided.

Irregular astigmatism resulting from a refractive surgical procedure may compromise the ultimate visual outcome following cataract surgery. To properly counsel the patient preoperatively, the surgeon should attempt to estimate the degree to which irregular astigmatism is responsible for decreased visual function. This can be accomplished by using a hard contact lens to mask the astigmatism while performing an overrefraction.

Choosing the lens implant power for a cataract patient after refractive surgery can be difficult because the effective corneal power cannot be accurately assessed from the keratometric readings. For further discussion, see Chapter 8, Primary Intraocular Lens Implantation in Adults, IOL Power Determination.

Developmental Abnormalities

When considering surgery in an adult with an acquired cataract and a developmentally abnormal eye, the ophthalmologist must first determine the visual potential of the eye. A review of medical records may reveal the patient's visual acuity and/or visual fields before the development of cataract. After determining when the cataract developed, the clinician can question the patient specifically about visual tasks that have subsequently become more difficult. Potential acuity testing may be helpful. The clinician must be reasonably certain that the reduction in visual function is a result of the cataract and not a consequence of another ocular problem such as amblyopia or retinal disease. The presence of a dense afferent pupillary defect and/or the absence of entoptic phenomena or color discrimination suggests a poor prognosis for recovering visual function. Nevertheless, improvement in visual acuity from hand motions or counting fingers to 20/200 can significantly improve the quality of life for a low vision patient. If the lens opacity interferes with the fundus examination, ultrasonography should be performed to rule out retinal detachment, staphyloma, or a mass lesion in the posterior segment. Ultrasonography can also be used to assess the size of the globe.

Next, the clinician should evaluate how well the eye will tolerate cataract surgery. A small cornea has less endothelial reserve because it has fewer endothelial cells. By performing pachymetry in the morning, when the cornea is thickest, the surgeon can identify a cornea that is likely to decompensate postoperatively.

Eyes with abnormal angle structures are at greater risk for glaucoma. Even if the patient has no history of glaucoma, elevated IOP can develop postoperatively. If the patient has already been diagnosed with elevated IOP that requires multiple medications for control, the physician should consider preoperative laser trabeculoplasty or combining cataract surgery with glaucoma filtering surgery (see Ocular Conditions, Glaucoma, Cataract Surgery Combined With Glaucoma). Preoperative evaluation in this setting should include a visual field, if possible. Glaucomatous optic nerve damage may be difficult to assess when the discs are anomalous.

In the presence of *iris coloboma* (Fig 10-5A), zonular dehiscence may occur in the area of exposure. Preoperative detection of this condition prepares the surgeon and the patient for an increased risk of vitreous loss. A capsular tension ring with coloboma diaphragm (Fig 10-5B) may help to reduce the risk of vitreous loss.

Posterior polar cataracts, which are often bilateral and inherited in an autosomal dominant pattern, increase the risk for intraoperative posterior capsular rupture and require careful patient selection and preoperative counseling. To minimize this complication, the least amount of stress possible must be placed on the posterior capsule. Retrobulbar or peribulbar anesthetic can be used to prevent ocular movement that could result in posterior vitreous pressure. Also, throughout the procedure, hypotony must be avoided to prevent vitreous pressure on the posterior capsule. Viscoelastic can be used to maintain the anterior chamber. Hydrodelineation should be performed, but hydrodissection should be avoided. Endophacoemulsification helps to maintain coverage over the possible posterior capsule defect. Removing the peripheral epinucleus should be done first, with removal of the core nucleus left until the end. Epinuclear removal is the most likely time for the posterior capsule to rupture. Lowering the infusion bottle will decrease

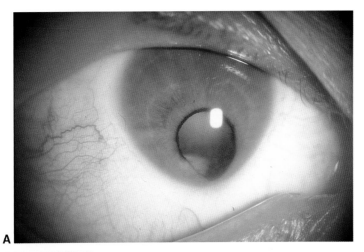

A

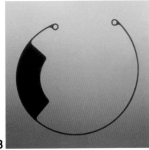

B

Figure 10-5 **A**, Coloboma of the iris with nuclear cataract. Instability of zonular support may be present in the area of the iris defect. Preoperative evaluation to identify associated posterior segment abnormalities is important in determining visual potential. **B**, A capsular tension ring with coloboma diaphragm. *(Part A courtesy of Robert S. Feder, MD; part B courtesy of Morcher GmbH, Stuttgart.)*

the pressure on the posterior capsule. Attempts to polish the posterior capsule may result in capsular rupture.

Retinopathy of prematurity is associated with nuclear cataracts that can be denser than anticipated for the patient's age. These patients are often highly myopic but generally do not have a long axial length. If they have undergone retinal cryotreatment or retinal detachment repair, they may have associated zonular laxity.

Nanophthalmos is a rare condition in which the eye is pathologically small (Fig 10-6). The ratio of lens volume to eye volume is higher than normal in these eyes, which also have shallow anterior chambers, narrow angles, and thickened sclerae. Intraocular surgery is generally hazardous because of the risk of intraoperative or postoperative uveal effusion. This is another condition in which small-incision surgery is clearly indicated.

The surgeon must decide if and when an IOL should be inserted in eyes whose size or proportions differ substantially from normal. For example, standard size IOLs are not suitable for use in eyes with *microphthalmos* or *congenital anterior megalophthalmos* (Fig 10-7). In the latter condition, which is usually bilateral and inherited as an X-linked recessive trait, the anterior segment is disproportionately large compared to the rest of the eye. The cornea is usually larger than 13.0 mm in diameter. This condition is associated with corneal arcus, pigmentary dispersion syndrome, cataract, zonular dehiscence, dislocated lens, and high myopia. IOL manufacturers may be willing to adapt a standard lens implant design to meet the needs of an individual patient with an ocular develop-

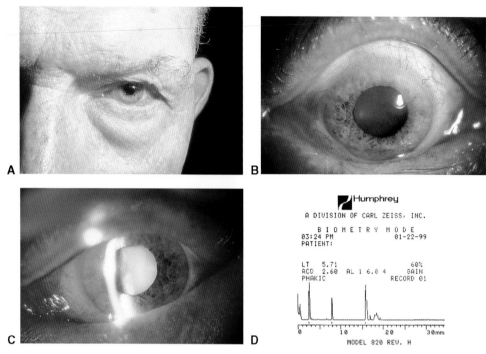

Figure 10-6 Nanophthalmos. **A**, Although this patient with nanophthalmos was phakic, he wore aphakic spectacles to correct high hyperopia. **B**, Corneal diameter was 10.5 mm. **C**, Preoperatively, the anterior chamber was somewhat shallow and a nuclear cataract was present. The best-corrected visual acuity was 20/200. **D**, Ultrasound axial length measurement was 16 mm, and biometry suggested the need for a 48 D lens implant. A 45 D PMMA lens, the highest power commercially available at the time of publication, was implanted. A piggyback IOL approach is perhaps a less suitable alternative in such a small eye. *(Photographs courtesy of Robert S. Feder, MD.)*

mental abnormality, but it may take several months to obtain such a lens and may require permission from the hospital's institutional review board.

Choosing the proper lens power may be difficult if the cornea is abnormally flat—for example, in a patient with *sclerocornea* (Fig 10-8). The average keratometry value for the cornea depicted in the figure is 30.0 D, compared to the normal average of 42.5 D. This condition is usually sporadic, and in addition to the flat corneal contour, it is characterized by opacification that can involve the entire cornea or just the periphery. Abnormalities of the iris and anterior chamber angle may also be associated.

It may also be a challenge to determine IOL power in a *keratoconus* patient because the cornea is abnormally steep and irregular astigmatism is usually present. If the patient successfully wears a contact lens, the clinician should explain that contact lens wear will most likely still be needed postoperatively, despite IOL implantation. If the patient is young, the keratoconus may continue to progress until penetrating keratoplasty (PK) is required. In that case, a lens exchange or piggyback IOL procedure may be performed at the time of the PK to adjust the refractive power to the anticipated postoperative corneal contour. A piggyback IOL can also be performed after the cornea is stable.

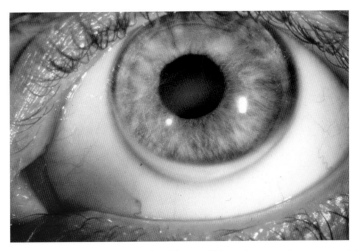

Figure 10-7 Anterior megalophthalmos. In this condition, the anterior segment is dispropor-tionately large in proportion to the rest of the eye, and the cornea is usually greater than 13.0 mm in diameter. The diameter of the cornea shown here is 15.0 mm.

If a *posterior staphyloma* is present, an accurate axial length measurement may be difficult to obtain.

Depending on the contour and size of the cornea and the presence or absence of nystagmus, an aphakic contact lens may or may not be a suitable alternative to an IOL. A binocular patient who cannot use a contact lens and whose cataractous eye is not suitable for IOL insertion may not be a candidate for cataract surgery. However, in a binocular patient with a mature cataract, even the aphakic state may provide enough improvement in peripheral vision to justify the surgery. A monocular aphakic patient could be offered aphakic spectacles.

When surgery on a developmentally abnormal eye is being planned, it is especially important for the surgeon to carefully discuss the risks and the benefits and to encourage the patient to participate in the decision-making process. The surgeon should alert the operating room staff about the nature of the case so that potentially necessary equipment is readily available. In general, it is wise in this surgical situation to expect the unexpected.

Increased Risk of Expulsive Hemorrhage

Among the risk factors for expulsive choroidal hemorrhage are advanced age, uncon-trolled glaucoma, myopia, choroidal sclerosis, arterial hypertension, generalized arterio-sclerosis, anticoagulation therapy or bleeding diathesis, recent trauma or surgery with active inflammation, prolonged hypotony, and previous expulsive hemorrhage in the fellow eye with cataract surgery. Although it is impossible to control all of these risk factors, preparing the patient and surgical team for the possibility of expulsive hemor-rhage is helpful. Expulsive choroidal hemorrhage can occur under general or local an-esthesia (regardless of whether epinephrine is used with the local retrobulbar anesthetic). It may occur with general anesthesia when the patient is bucking or coughing from the

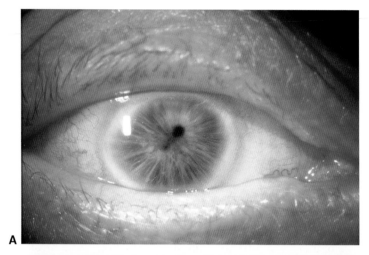

A

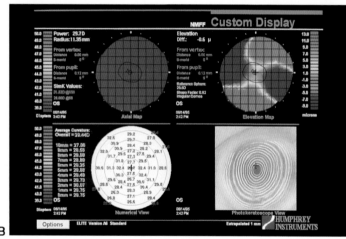

B

Figure 10-8 A, Sclerocornea (cornea plana). Although sometimes inherited, this condition usu-ally occurs sporadically. It is characterized by a flat corneal contour and opacification that may involve the periphery of, or the entire, cornea. The average keratometry value of the cornea illustrated here is 30.0 D (normal corneas average 42.5 D). Lens implant power can be difficult to determine when the cornea is flatter than the limit of measurement with the keratometer. **B**, A corneal power map from a sclerocornea patient shows markedly flat cornea with simulated keratometry readings of less than 30.0 D. *(Photographs courtesy of Robert S. Feder, MD.)*

endotracheal tube if the level of anesthesia lightens, although with modern anesthesia techniques this complication is less likely to occur.

Phacoemulsification surgery provides several advantages to the high-risk patient. The small incision can be closed rapidly if hemorrhage occurs. The technique minimizes the time that the eye is hypotonous and helps reduce the wide fluctuations in IOP that can occur with some irrigation/aspiration systems. In general, the overall operating time is significantly less for small-incision surgery. Nevertheless, small-incision surgery cannot entirely prevent the occurrence of choroidal hemorrhage.

If IOP is high, the surgeon should avoid rapid decompression of the eye when making the initial incision. A compression device such as a Honan balloon or gentle digital massage may be used to lower IOP before the eye is surgically opened. In addition, the conjunctiva can be opened more posteriorly than normal and an area of sclera prepared for a sclerostomy, if needed, in the event of a hemorrhage. Meticulous attention to wound closure is essential: expulsive hemorrhage can occur postoperatively as well as intra-operatively. In the perioperative period, the patient should be cautioned to avoid Valsalva maneuvers.

Glaucoma

Management

Glaucoma patients who use miotic eyedrops may experience visual symptoms from cataract prematurely because of their small pupils. If miotic medications can be withdrawn or another type of therapy substituted without jeopardizing IOP control, visual function may improve even without cataract surgery. Current glaucoma medications have lessened the need for miotics, and this problem is not as prevalent as in past years. Phakic patients are generally more responsive to argon laser trabeculoplasty, which may provide IOP control without the use of miotic agents.

When the patient is troubled by the cataract, and either miotic agents cannot be withdrawn or the patient has permanent miosis from long-term miotic use, cataract surgery is usually required. Surgical options include cataract surgery alone, combined cataract/filtering surgery, or staged procedures of filtering surgery followed by cataract surgery at a later time. Cataract surgery alone may be appropriate if the IOP is well controlled with medical therapy, the patient is compliant and tolerates the medications, and the glaucomatous optic nerve damage is not severe. Small-incision cataract surgery with posterior chamber lens implantation has been shown to restore visual function without compromising glaucoma control. In some glaucoma patients, IOP control improves after cataract extraction, obviating the need for glaucoma surgery. This improvement may result either from correction of a phacomorphic component to the obstruction of aqueous outflow or from a change in aqueous production. Small-incision cataract surgery by the clear corneal approach is advantageous because it minimizes conjunctival damage, an important consideration if future filtering surgery may be needed.

If the glaucoma patient has a borderline cataract and could easily tolerate a second procedure, a staged approach can be considered. Patients should be advised, however, that, as a result of inflammation, lens trauma, flat anterior chamber, hypotony, or corticosteroid use, their cataracts may progress more quickly after glaucoma filtering surgery. In addition, the function of the glaucoma filter may be compromised by later cataract surgery.

Cataracts and other opacities, including corneal dystrophic changes, can cause abnormalities of visual fields. The clinician who fails to consider the effect of abnormal media may underestimate the visual potential of the eye. Other factors, such as the appearance of the disc and the reactivity of the pupil, must also be evaluated when possible. (Figure 10-9 demonstrates visual fields in a glaucoma patient before and after combined cataract and penetrating keratoplasty surgery.)

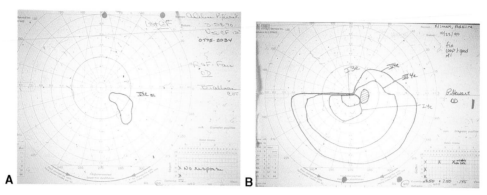

Figure 10-9 Cataracts, as well as other media opacities, can markedly reduce the visual field. **A**, The preoperative Goldmann visual field in a 78-year-old glaucoma patient with Fuchs corneal dystrophy and cataract. **B**, The Goldmann visual field following penetrating keratoplasty with ECCE and insertion of a posterior chamber lens. *(Photographs courtesy of Robert S. Feder, MD.)*

Stank T, Feitl ME, Krupin T. Cataract surgery in glaucoma. In: Weinstock FJ, ed. *Management and Care of the Cataract Patient.* Boston: Blackwell Scientific Publications; 1992:160–170.

Complications of cataract surgery in the glaucoma patient

Postoperative inflammation is frequently more severe in a glaucomatous eye, with more serious consequences. The degree of inflammation is a function of both the preoperative ocular condition and the amount of intraocular manipulation during surgery. In addition, the use of strong miotics such as echothiophate iodide (Phospholine) can be associated with an exuberant postoperative inflammatory reaction. The use of latanoprost (Xalatan), a topical prostaglandin preparation, can also be associated with increased postoperative inflammation.

Postoperative *IOP increases* after cataract surgery occur more commonly and to higher levels in patients with glaucoma. Two thirds of glaucomatous eyes have a pressure rise of more than 7–10 mm Hg on the first postoperative day. Viscoelastic agents commonly used in cataract surgery can easily block an already compromised trabecular meshwork, even when the material is aspirated. Blood, pigment, inflammatory material, and lens cortex can also obstruct outflow and contribute to a postoperative pressure elevation. Thus, glaucoma patients should be followed closely in the immediate postsurgical period in order to detect and manage increases in IOP.

The clinician should consider combined cataract and filtering surgery if the eye will not tolerate a significant pressure elevation or if the patient will not be able to tolerate the medications needed to obtain pressure control. (For more detailed discussion, see Ocular Conditions, Glaucoma, Cataract Surgery Combined With Glaucoma Filtering Surgery.)

The glaucoma patient is at higher risk of postoperative *cystoid macular edema (CME).* Cystoid macular edema may occur more frequently in glaucoma patients because of their tendency toward greater postoperative inflammation. Moreover, some of the medications used by glaucoma patients, including dipivefrin (Propine) and possibly latanoprost, increase the risk of postoperative CME. Although CME is usually reversible, its resolution may take months. Patients should be warned that CME can slow their process of post-operative visual rehabilitation. Topical NSAIDs may be helpful. (For further discussion of CME and its treatment, see Cystoid Macular Edema in Chapter 9.)

Intraoperative *vitreous loss* in the glaucoma patient may result from loose zonular fibers, and thus, zonular status should be assessed preoperatively. Signs indicating lack of zonular support include asymmetric anterior chamber depth, iridodonesis, irido-dialysis, phacodonesis, or tilting of the lens. Loose zonular fibers are seen in glaucoma associated with exfoliation syndrome or trauma. The condition can also result from inadequate intraoperative management of the small pupil combined with the external pressure applied in expressing the nucleus. In conventional ECCE with reduced zonular support, removing the nucleus with a lens loop can sometimes be helpful in reducing the chance of vitreous loss. Phacoemulsification also decreases the risk of vitreous loss because no external pressure is required to remove the nucleus. If vitreous loss occurs in the presence of a functioning filter, the vitreous can clog the sclerostomy. A careful vitrectomy is required to ensure that such an obstruction does not occur.

The *small pupil* can be managed in several ways. Traditionally, a peripheral iridectomy and posterior synechialysis were performed, and a radial iridotomy connected the iri-dectomy with the pupil. Inferior, lateral, and/or medial sphincterotomies would be added as needed to provide adequate access to the lens. Following IOL insertion, the iridotomy could be repaired. Contemporary techniques include creating multiple tiny, equally spaced sphincterotomies using intraocular scissors. Permanent mydriasis can be avoided if the cuts do not extend through the sphincter into the iris stroma. Alternatively, the iris sphincter can be stretched using instruments inserted through paracentesis sites, engaging the iris at the pupil margin, and slowly and gently stretching the sphincter. Hemorrhage at the pupil margin is not uncommon. Viscoelastic injected intracamerally can further dilate the pupil. If dilation is inadequate, the iris sphincter can be stretched in the axis 90° from the first procedure. Other devices to stretch the pupil are available.

The self-retaining flexible iris retractor is a microsurgical innovation that allows adequate enlargement of the pupil without iris incision (Fig 10-10). The retractors can be used even with topical/intracameral anesthesia. Each retractor is inserted through a separate stab incision in the peripheral cornea. Near the phacoemulsification wound, the retractors should be placed approximately 60° apart to facilitate insertion of the handpiece tip without engaging the iris. Distal to the phacoemulsification wound, the retractors should be placed approximately 90° apart. The retractors can easily be removed following IOL insertion. However, when cataract surgery is combined with glaucoma filtering sur-gery, a peripheral iridectomy is usually performed at the sclerostomy site to prevent occlusion by the iris.

Cataract surgery following a glaucoma filtering procedure

The ophthalmologist can perform cataract surgery following a glaucoma filtering procedure in several different ways. Small-incision phacoemulsification surgery should be used in this setting unless contraindicated. Compared to ECCE, the smaller wound is more secure, the surgery is generally less traumatic, and visual rehabilitation is more rapid.

If the glaucoma filter is no longer functioning but is still needed, cataract extraction can be done at the site of the existing filter, and the bleb can be revised at the same time.

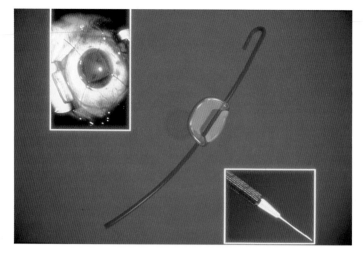

Figure 10-10 One type of flexible iris retractor. *(Courtesy of Grieshaber and Company, Inc.)*

Operating at a familiar position is advantageous; however, revising the bleb may be less successful than performing a combined cataract extraction and filtering surgery at a virgin site. If a new filtering site is selected, cataract surgery can be performed through the new site or through a temporal clear corneal approach.

If the glaucoma filter is still functioning, every effort should be made to protect it. It is estimated that 30%–50% of glaucoma filters fail after cataract surgery when the conjunctiva has been manipulated. Clear corneal phacoemulsification through a temporal approach is the preferred technique in the presence of a functioning bleb because it reduces conjunctival trauma and minimizes corneal astigmatism.

In-the-bag posterior chamber lens implantation is the preferred technique for several reasons. For one, optimal lens centration is more reliably obtained. Further, this technique reduces the chances of capture of the optic within the pupil, postoperative inflammation, and vitreous herniation through a posterior capsulotomy. In addition, in the event of a shallow or flat chamber postoperatively, the cornea is probably better protected if the IOL is behind the iris and within the capsule.

Cataract surgery combined with glaucoma filtering surgery

Glaucoma filtering surgery combined with cataract surgery is recommended for the patient with glaucoma and cataract under the following circumstances:

- visually significant cataract and maximal tolerated glaucoma medications
- visually significant cataract and poor compliance with required glaucoma medications
- visually significant cataract with moderate to severe glaucomatous visual field loss
- visually significant cataract with severe glaucomatous damage to the optic nerve, which could not withstand a postoperative IOP increase
- visually significant cataract together with inadequate bleb function

- visually significant cataract in a glaucoma patient unable to tolerate multiple procedures
- even if not otherwise visually significant, a cataract that prevents adequate visual fields or optic disc evaluation

Many techniques have been described for combined cataract and glaucoma filtering surgery. Trabeculectomy and guarded posterior lip sclerostomy are most commonly used. Phacoemulsification is preferred over conventional extracapsular cataract surgery in this setting. The rate of bleb survival is more than 3 times higher after combined procedures using phacoemulsification than after trabeculectomy and extracapsular surgery (62% versus 20%). Finally, the risks of postoperative hyphema, fibrinous iritis, hypotony, and choroidal detachment are less with phacoemulsification.

Shingleton BJ, Jacobson LM, Kuperwaser MC. Comparison of combined cataract and glaucoma surgery using planned extracapsular and phacoemulsificiation techniques. *Ophthalmic Surg Lasers.* 1995;26:414–419.

Small-incision cataract surgery can be completed under a partial-thickness scleral flap at the site of the trabeculectomy or through a separate incision. The temporal clear corneal approach to cataract surgery combined with trabeculectomy is gaining popularity. However, the long-term advantage of the so-called *two-site combined procedure* is not yet proven.

Failure of the filter is more likely when the patient is young or has a darkly pigmented iris, a history of iritis, conjunctival scarring, or a previously failed filter. Such patients may require antimetabolite therapy at the time of surgery, which may reduce the likelihood of poor filtration caused by scarring of the conjunctiva or the sclerostomy. Mitomycin C is currently the preferred antiproliferative agent. (See also BCSC Section 10, *Glaucoma.*)

Balyeat HD. Cataract surgery in the glaucoma patient. Part 1: a cataract surgeon's perspective. *Focal Points: Clinical Modules for Ophthalmologists.* San Francisco: American Academy of Ophthalmology; 1998, module 3.

Skuta GL. Cataract surgery in the glaucoma patient. Part 2: a glaucoma surgeon's perspective. *Focal Points: Clinical Modules for Ophthalmologists.* San Francisco: American Academy of Ophthalmology; 1998, module 4.

High Refractive Error

The crystalline lens adds about 15–20 D of refractive power to the eye. Individuals with a refractive error greater than –6.00 or +6.00 D have reduced visual function. Spectacle lenses can be thick and heavy. The image size through a high-minus lens is minified and that through a high-plus lens is magnified. Peripheral vision is reduced through either a high-plus or a high-minus lens. Much of this disability can be eliminated if the patient can tolerate contact lenses. Further, when the patient with high myopia develops a significant cataract, surgery with or without an IOL can greatly improve visual function.

Surgical considerations in high myopia

At the start of phacoemulsification in a patient with high myopia, the anterior chamber may deepen dramatically, making nuclear sculpting difficult. It is advisable to lower the irrigation bottle and increase the flow rate before placing the phaco tip in the eye. When possible, the patient should receive an IOL, which can act as a barrier to the forward movement of vitreous if a capsulotomy becomes necessary. A minus-power IOL is available for those patients who would have significant residual myopia with even the lowest plus-power IOL. Foldable IOLs are now available in minus powers in both silicone and acrylic material. Even uncomplicated cataract surgery in patients with high myopia increases the risk of retinal detachment. Silicone IOLs with an open posterior capsule develop condensation that compromises the retinal surgeon's view if a pars plana vitrectomy is required; therefore, their use is relatively contraindicated for these patients.

Surgical considerations in high hyperopia

The cataract patient with high hyperopia often has a shallow anterior chamber and is more prone to uveal prolapse and iris trauma than is the patient with myopia. Phacoemulsification can be facilitated by deepening the anterior chamber by using extra viscoelastic and raising the irrigation bottle prior to insertion of the phaco tip. The risk of iris prolapse can be reduced by creating a slightly more anterior wound. The hyperopic eye may have a smaller-than-average corneal diameter, making it more susceptible to complications from corneal trauma associated with cataract surgery. To protect the cornea, particularly when a more anterior wound has been created, the surgeon should minimize intraocular manipulation.

Clear lens extraction

Clear lens extraction has been advocated for the correction of high myopia and high hyperopia, given the success of phacoemulsification surgery. The purported advantages of this technique over other refractive surgery techniques include sparing the central visual axis from corneal manipulation, preservation of Bowman's layer and the normal corneal contour, and the familiarity of most cataract surgeons with the technique. However, the improvement in visual function must be weighed against the risks. For example, the risk of retinal detachment after clear lens extraction is estimated to be 1.1% per year in the patient with high myopia. Further, if Nd:YAG laser posterior capsulotomy becomes necessary, it may increase the risk of retinal detachment. In addition, standard IOL power formulas are less predictable when larger degrees of refractive error correction are attempted. This refractive procedure is used more often for correction of moderate hyperopia. Other potential complications of clear lens extraction include endophthalmitis, corneal decompensation, glaucoma, hemorrhage, IOL dislocation, and ptosis. A consent form specific for this procedure should be considered. The controversy over the risk–benefit ratio of refractive lensectomy continues to be influenced by the development of alternative surgical methods for the correction of high degrees of refractive error.

Colin J, Robinet A, Cochener B. Retinal detachment after clear lens extraction for high myopia: seven-year follow-up. *Ophthalmology*. 1999;106:2281–2285.

Hypotony

In general, severe ocular hypotony (pre-phthisis) is a prognostic indicator of poor visual potential. An evaluation of the cause of the hypotony should be undertaken preoperatively. If the view of the posterior segment is inadequate, ultrasonography can be helpful. Reversible causes of hypotony, such as iritis with ciliary body shutdown, should be controlled before cataract surgery. The presence of a cyclodialysis cleft or retinal detachment may necessitate a separate corrective procedure or a more extensive procedure combined with cataract surgery. Chronic hypotony can result in shortened axial length and choroidal thickening, which can make IOL power selection more complicated and less predictable. Irreversible hypotony is a contraindication for cataract surgery.

Uveitis

Chronic recurring intraocular inflammation and the corticosteroid therapy used to treat it are both risk factors for the development of cataract. When the cataract becomes significant, the surgeon must determine the relative contributions of the cataract and the coexisting ocular disease to the reduction in visual function. Cystoid macular edema, when associated, can usually be seen with fluorescein angiography or angioscopy. Patients with uveitis should be warned that their visual prognosis is guarded because of potential postoperative complications such as corneal edema; exacerbation of intraocular inflammation, glaucoma, or hypotony; choroidal effusion; or macular edema. If the patient has not already had an appropriate workup to determine the cause of uveitis, it should be done prior to planning surgery.

The risk of complications can be reduced if the inflammation is well controlled prior to the surgery and if postoperative inflammation is treated aggressively. In most cases, these patients should be pretreated with frequent topical or oral steroids and maintained on intensive therapy in the perioperative period. Topical or systemic cyclosporine may be indicated in selected patients.

Historically, IOLs were strictly contraindicated in uveitis patients. Since the technique of ECCE with intracapsular posterior chamber IOL became widely adopted, however, this contraindication has become less absolute, and the widespread use of small-incision phacoemulsification surgery has made IOL placement in uveitis patients routine. Certain types of uveitis, including Fuchs heterochromic iridocyclitis, quiescent recurrent acute iritis, and inactive posterior uveitis, may do well with IOLs. A relatively small, prospective, randomized study of IOL insertion in uveitis cases concluded that patients with chronic iridocyclitis or pars planitis do well with lens implants but that visual acuity may be better without an implant. An IOL with a PMMA or acrylic optic may be preferable to a flexible silicone IOL in the uveitis patient.

Foster CS. Cataract surgery in the patient with uveitis. *Focal Points: Clinical Modules for Ophthalmologists.* San Francisco: American Academy of Ophthalmology; 1994, module 4.

Tessler HH, Farber MD. Intraocular lens implantation versus no intraocular lens implantation in patients with chronic iridocyclitis and pars planitis. A randomized prospective study. *Ophthalmology.* 1993;100:1206–1209.

Retinal Disease

Macular degeneration

The coexistence of macular degeneration and cataract can present a challenge to the surgeon attempting to predict the outcome of planned cataract surgery. A review of old records may help to uncover the patient's visual acuity before the development of the cataract but after the macular disease was present. As a rule, functional testing using potential acuity evaluation techniques is a better predictor of surgical outcome than is macular appearance. Good performance on potential acuity testing is encouraging; however, a poor performance is not necessarily an accurate predictor of surgical outcome. Another test of macular function that may be helpful is a macular photostress test (see Measurements of Visual Function in Chapter 7).

Whenever cataract surgery is planned in the presence of macular degeneration, the patient must be forewarned that the prognosis is guarded. Surgery is indicated if the cataract interferes with a detailed examination of the macula, hindering the diagnosis and treatment of a subretinal neovascular membrane.

Retinitis pigmentosa

Retinitis pigmentosa is often associated with posterior subcapsular cataracts. Dense cataracts can constrict the already diminished visual field, and disabling glare can further reduce visual function. The assessment of visual potential in patients with retinitis pigmentosa may be difficult. Favorable results of potential acuity testing may be misleading. The macula should be examined preoperatively to rule out the presence of CME or other abnormalities in this region of the retina. The patient's subjective complaints of decreased vision coinciding with the development of cataract, along with the surgeon's appreciation of the degree of opacity, are often good indications that surgery will improve visual function.

Following pars plana vitrectomy

Cataract is a common complication of phakic pars plana vitrectomy. The cataract induced is most often nuclear, with central distortion of the red reflex. The visual significance of the cataract may not be appreciated by slit-lamp appearance. Some affected eyes benefit from cataract extraction and IOL implantation. The lack of a stabilizing influence from the vitreous body makes the posterior capsule unusually mobile, dictating modifications in surgical technique. Zonular integrity may be diminished because of prior surgery. During phacoemulsification, the anterior chamber may become quite deep. It is recommended that the irrigation bottle be lowered and the flow rate increased prior to placing the phaco tip in the eye. Attempting phacoemulsification in an extremely deep anterior chamber places further stress on the zonular fibers, but a large capsulorrhexis will allow prolapse of the nucleus during hydrodissection for iris plane phaco chop. If an extracapsular surgical technique is selected because of a large brunescent nucleus, attempts to express the nucleus by external pressure on the inferior limbus are generally unsuccessful and may cause zonular dehiscence. Alternatively, after capsulorrhexis, the nucleus can be hydrodissected from its cortical attachments, elevated with a spatula or cannula, and removed by means of a lens loop or irrigating vectis.

Trauma

Cataract may be an early or late manifestation of ocular trauma (see Chapter 5). Rupture of the lens capsule generally leads to rapid hydration of the lens cortex, causing a milky white cataract to form. Lens protein may leak into the aqueous and vitreous and may cause uveitis and/or glaucoma. When cortical material is noted in the anterior chamber, the cataract should be removed promptly. A mature cataract obscures the fundus and interferes with the diagnosis and treatment of injuries in the posterior segment. Release of lens material may produce a secondary glaucoma that is difficult to treat and can mask or mimic infectious endophthalmitis. Any of these conditions may necessitate the removal of a cataract acutely after ocular trauma. Care must be taken to rule out the possibility of fibrin covering a clear lens. Children are especially likely after trauma to form fibrin in the aqueous that can masquerade as cataract.

A slowly progressive cataract should be followed while intraocular inflammation is being controlled. Slowly progressive or stationary cataracts should be removed only if visually significant for the patient. A patient with a dense cataract and a history of ocular trauma should be evaluated to determine the potential for visual recovery following surgery. In addition to reviewing the complete history and available records, the surgeon should look for gross visual field defects, afferent pupillary defect, sphincter tears or angle abnormalities, elevated or abnormally low IOP, and ultrasound evidence of posterior segment pathology.

Many factors must be considered in planning cataract extraction after recent trauma, as discussed in the following sections.

Visualization

Corneal laceration and/or edema may impair the surgeon's ability to safely remove lens material and, thus, may indicate the need for an open-sky approach. Hemorrhage can occur during lens removal and further interfere with visualization. If the hemorrhage cannot be controlled and visualization is difficult, use of air and/or viscoelastics may be helpful. If visualization remains insufficient, the eye should be closed to allow an adequate clot to form.

Inflammation

During the acute phase of ocular trauma, fibrin rapidly forms membranes on the iris that can cause synechiae, pupil seclusion, and distortion of intraocular structures. Gentle sweeping of the posterior synechiae may allow the pupil to dilate, but if it does not, pupilloplasty may be necessary. A peripheral iridectomy is important in this setting in order to prevent postoperative pupillary block. Inflamed uveal tissue is fragile, and bleeding frequently occurs during surgery. Viscoelastics should be used liberally to protect damaged corneal endothelium and possibly to improve the view of anterior segment structures. Postoperative IOP elevation may occur even when viscoelastic removal has been attempted. Use of cycloplegics and intensive topical and possibly oral steroid therapy are essential to control the perioperative inflammation.

Retained Foreign Matter

Depending on the type of injury, the ophthalmologist may suspect that an intraocular foreign body is present. If the media are sufficiently clear, indirect ophthalmoscopy is an excellent way to look for a retained foreign body; if the view is inadequate, CT scan or ultrasound can be helpful. MRI should not be used if there is a possibility of a metallic foreign body because the foreign body could be dislodged by the magnetic force of the procedure. Significant cataract in the presence of retained foreign matter in the posterior chamber may be handled via a pars plana approach or an anterior approach (with lens implantation if indicated) followed by a pars plana vitrectomy and foreign body removal. Intracameral foreign bodies may be easier to see at the slit lamp than at the operating microscope, making removal more difficult. In addition, irrigating solutions can dislodge a foreign body from its preoperative position.

Damage to Other Ocular Tissues

The iris is frequently disrupted when trauma to the lens occurs. Dialyses may be repaired by suturing the iris root to the scleral spur. Sphincter ruptures rarely need repair unless clinically significant papillary distortion has resulted. Vitreous is generally disturbed by trauma that ruptures the posterior lens capsule, and careful removal of vitreous from the anterior segment improves the prognosis for the trauma surgery. Large amounts of lens material can become sequestered behind the iris; iris retraction and removal of this material should be attempted to allow a clearer view of the peripheral retina. Cataract extraction may be necessary to allow adequate visualization if a retinal detachment occurs early or late in the course.

Zonular Dehiscence With Lens Subluxation or Dislocation

Commonly encountered causes of zonular incompetence include exfoliation syndrome and trauma. Congenital and developmental disorders such as Marfan syndrome and inborn errors of metabolism are less common causes of inadequate zonular support. Iridodonesis may be the initial clinical sign indicating zonular disruption. Posterior dislocations without lens rupture may require only observation. Frequently, some zonular fibers remain intact, tethering the lens in the anterior vitreous. When the patient is examined upright at the slit lamp, the lens may seem easily accessible for extraction, but when the patient is positioned for surgery, the lens may fall back out of reach. Thus, it is helpful to examine the patient in the supine position preoperatively.

Zonular incompetence not suspected preoperatively may present intraoperatively by decentration of the lens and capsular bag or vitreous prolapse into the anterior chamber, with loss of efficient nuclear removal (Fig 10-11). Phacoemulsification can sometimes be used to extract a cataract in the presence of limited zonular support. A generous capsulorrhexis will facilitate nucleus extraction; however, the surgeon should be careful to avoid extending the capsular tear into the area of zonular fiber insertion on the anterior capsule. Reducing the flow rate helps to decrease both anterior chamber turbulence and the risk of vitreous prolapse through the zonular dehiscence. Lowering the bottle height reduces the chance of a very deep anterior chamber, which can further stress the zonular fibers. The surgeon must adjust both bottle height and flow rate so that aspiration can still be done efficiently.

A traumatic cataract is usually soft and can be aspirated through the large aspiration port of the phaco tip, especially in a young patient. Viscoelastic tamponade of vitreous can be used for areas of zonular incompetence. If a nuclear cataract was present before the trauma, sufficient ultrasound power should be used to emulsify the nucleus without moving it excessively. If vitreous has migrated into the anterior chamber, anterior vitrectomy should be performed before starting phacoemulsification or cortical aspiration to avoid vitreous aspiration with resulting retinal traction.

If there is not enough capsular support to allow phacoemulsification, an *endocapsular tension ring* (Fig 10-12) can be inserted into the capsular bag. This device provides adequate support for nucleus and cortical removal, as well as for in-the-bag IOL insertion. If a capsular tension ring is not available and zonular support is sufficient for in-the-bag IOL placement, a 3-piece IOL with the haptics placed in the area of zonular weakness helps prevent capsular contraction.

When the nucleus is markedly subluxed and vitreous fills a substantial part of the anterior chamber, the surgeon should consider removing the cataract through a pars plana approach. Referral to a retina specialist is advisable if the surgeon is not skilled in this technique. An anterior chamber IOL or transclerally fixated posterior chamber lens may be necessary in case of inadequate capsular support for a posterior chamber IOL.

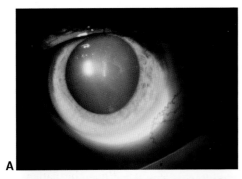

A

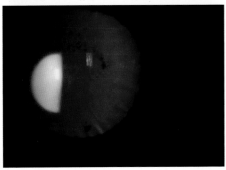

B

Figure 10-11 Patient with cataract and a distant history of trauma to the forehead. On slit-lamp examination, no movement of the lens was evident and the other eye was normal. **A,** Slit-lamp photo with diffuse illumination reveals pigment on the posterior aspect of the posterior capsule. **B,** Retroillumination reveals small transillumination defects in the iris as well as the pigmentary deposits on the posterior lens capsule. The red reflex highlights the anterior capsular wrinkling along the temporal side of the lens. This surface wrinkling of the anterior capsule was a preoperative suggestion of loose zonules that was confirmed at surgery. *(Photographs courtesy of Cynthia A. Bradford, MD.)*

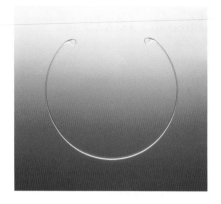

Figure 10-12 An endocapsular tension ring. *(Courtesy of Morcher GmbH, Stuttgart.)*

Lens Implantation

Primary IOL insertion can be considered when intraocular inflammation and hemorrhage are minimal and the view of anterior segment structures is good. Primary IOL insertion has the advantage of avoiding an additional operation, thus reducing the cost and risks associated with further intraocular surgery. The surgeon may nevertheless decide against primary IOL insertion in favor of aphakic contact lens use.

However, primary IOL insertion has some important disadvantages that should be considered preoperatively. Depending on the nature of the injury, some patients may be better served by having the IOL inserted in a secondary procedure. For example, less-than-optimal visualization may interfere with proper placement of the lens. Defects in the posterior capsule or zonular fibers that might not be recognized at the time of surgery can result in lens decentration or dislocation. The presence of an IOL may compromise a retinal surgeon's view of the peripheral retina and make repair more difficult in case of retinal detachment.

Further, if accurate biometry cannot be performed before primary IOL insertion, significant anisometropia may result. For example, corneal scarring resulting from a laceration can change the contour of the cornea at the visual axis and, ultimately, alter the IOL power required. A hard contact lens may be needed to mask irregular astigmatism, and the aphakic correction could be added to this lens. Finally, there is always a risk of endophthalmitis associated with perforating intraocular trauma, although the presence of an IOL does not seem to affect the ultimate prognosis.

Basic Texts

Lens and Cataract

Ajamian PC. *Pre- and Postoperative Care of the Cataract Patient*. Boston: Butterworth-Heinemann; 1993.

Apple DJ, Auffarth GU, Peng Q, et al. *Foldable Intraocular Lenses: Evolution, Clinicopathologic Correlations, and Complications*. Thorofare, NJ: Slack; 2000.

Bahadur GG, Sinskey RM. *Manual of Cataract Surgery*. 2nd ed. Boston: Butterworth-Heinemann; 1999.

Buratto L, Werner L, Zanini M, et al. *Phacoemulsification: Principles and Techniques*. 2nd ed. Thorofare, NJ: Slack; 2003.

Emery JM, Mcintyre DJ. *Extracapsular Cataract Surgery*. 2nd ed. St Louis: Mosby; 1990.

Fine IH. *Clear Corneal Lens Surgery*. Thorofare, NJ: Slack; 1999.

Gills JP. *Cataract Surgery: The State of the Art*. Thorofare, NJ: Slack; 1998.

Gills JP, Martin RG, Sanders DR, eds. *Sutureless Cataract Surgery: An Evolution Toward Minimally Invasive Technique*. Thorofare, NJ: Slack; 1992.

Harding J. *Cataract: Biochemistry, Epidemiology, and Pharmacology*. New York: Chapman & Hall; 1991.

Jaffe NS, Horwitz J. Lens and cataract. In: Podos SM, Yanoff M, eds. *Textbook of Ophthalmology*. St. Louis: Mosby; 1993.

Jaffe NS, Jaffe MS, Jaffe GF. *Cataract Surgery and Its Complications*. 6th ed. St Louis: Mosby; 1998.

Koch PS, Hoffman J. *Mastering Phacoemulsification: A Simplified Manual of Strategies for the Spring, Crack, and Stop and Chop Technique*. 4th ed. Thorofare, NJ: Slack; 1994.

Packard RBS, Kinnear FC. *Manual of Cataract and Intraocular Lens Surgery*. New York: Churchill Livingstone; 1991.

Retzlaff JA, Sanders DR, Kraff M. *Lens Implant Power Calculation: A Manual for Ophthalmologists and Biometrists*. 3rd ed. Thorofare, NJ: Slack; 1990.

Seibel BS. *Phacodynamics: Mastering the Tools and Techniques of Phacoemulsification Surgery*. 3rd ed. Thorofare, NJ: Slack; 1999.

Steinert RF, ed. *Cataract Surgery: Techniques, Complications, and Management*. 2nd ed. Philadelphia: Saunders; 2004.

Tasman W, Jaeger EA, eds. *Duane's Clinical Ophthalmology*. Philadelphia: Lippincott; 2001.

Tasman W, Jaeger EA, eds. *Duane's Foundations of Clinical Ophthalmology*. Philadelphia: Lippincott; 1992.

Weinstock FJ. *Management and Care of the Cataract Patient*. Boston: Blackwell Scientific Publications; 1992.

Young RW. *Age-Related Cataract*. New York: Oxford University Press; 1991.

Related Academy Materials

Focal Points: Clinical Modules for Ophthalmologists

Balyeat HD. Cataract surgery in the glaucoma patient. Part 1: a cataract surgeon's perspective (Module 3, 1998).

Byrnes GA. Evaluation of impaired visual acuity following cataract surgery (Module 6, 1996).

Fishkind WJ. The torn posterior capsule: prevention, recognition, and management (Module 4, 1999).

Foster CS. Cataract surgery in the patient with uveitis (Module 4, 1994).

Hoffer KJ. Modern IOL power calculations: avoiding error and planning for special circumstances (Module 12, 1999).

Koch DD. Cataract surgery following refractive surgery (Module 5, 2001).

Lane SS, Schwartz GS. IOL exchanges and secondary IOLs: surgical techniques (Module 1, 1998).

Maloney WF. Advances in small incision cataract surgery (Module 9, 2000).

Masket S. Cataract incision and closure (Module 3, 1995).

Nichamin LD. IOL update: new materials, designs, selection criteria, and insertional techniques (Module 11, 1999).

Rosenthal KJ. The capsular ring: indications and surgery (Module 7, 2002).

Ruttum MS. Childhood cataracts (Module 1, 1996).

Sanders DR, Retzlaff JA, Kraff MC. A-scan biometry and IOL calculations (Module 10, 1995).

Skuta GL. Cataract surgery in the glaucoma patient. Part 2: a glaucoma surgeon's perspective (Module 4, 1998).

Smiddy WE, Flynn HW Jr. Managing retained lens fragments and dislocated posterior chamber IOLs after cataract surgery (Module 7, 1996).

Stead SW, Bell SN. Ocular anesthesia (Module 3, 2001).

Wilson ME. Management of aphakia in children (Module 1, 1999).

Publications

Ford JG, Karp CL. *Cataract Surgery and Intraocular Lenses: A 21st-Century Perspective.* 2nd ed. (Ophthalmology Monograph 7, 2001).

Lane SS, Skuta GL, eds. *ProVision: Preferred Responses in Ophthalmology,* Series 3 (Self-Assessment Program, 1999).

Skuta GL, ed. *ProVision: Preferred Responses in Ophthalmology,* Series 2 (Self-Assessment Program, 1996).

Multimedia

Lane SL, Fine IH, Masket S, Steinert RF. *LEO Clinical Update Course on Cataract* (CD-ROM, 2003).

Continuing Ophthalmic Video Education

Al-Torbak AA. *Capsulorrhexis in Mature Cataract;* Dewey SH, Werner L, Apple DJ, et al. *Cortical Removal by J-Cannula Irrigation to Reduce Posterior Capsule Opacification;* Assi AC, Lacey A, Aylward B. *Basic Properties of Intraocular Gases;* Busin M, Arffa RC. *Deep Suturing Techniques for Penetrating Keratoplasty;* Teichmann KD, Al-Rajhi AA. *Maximum Depth Lamellar Keratoplasty for Keratoconus With Anwar's Big Bubble* (2001).

Lane SS, Koch DD. *Current Techniques in Phacoemulsification* (1995, Revised 1999).

Mead MD, Steinert RF. *Scleral Suture Fixation of Posterior Chamber Intraocular Lenses* (1997).

Osher RH. *Challenging Cases in Cataract Surgery* (2001).

Osher RH. *Complications During Phacoemulsification* (1999).

Osher RH. *More Challenging Cases in Cataract Surgery* (2001).

Preferred Practice Patterns

Preferred Practice Patterns Committee, Anterior Segment Panel. *Cataract in the Adult Eye* (2001).

Ophthalmic Technology Assessments

Ophthalmic Technology Assessment Committee. *Intraocular Lens Implantation in the Absence of Ocular Support* (2003).

Complementary Therapy Assessments

Complementary Therapy Task Force. *Antioxidant Vitamin and Mineral Supplements and Cataract Prevention and Progression* (2002).

Slide-Script

Fong DS. *Eye Care for the Elderly* (Eye Care Skills for the Primary Care Physician Series, 1999).

Specialty Clinical Update Online

Packer M, Fine IH, Hoffman RS. *Pulse and Burst Mode Phacoemulsification.* Module 1, 2003.

To order any of these materials, please call the Academy's Customer Service number at (415) 561-8540, or order online at www.aao.org.

Credit Reporting Form

Basic and Clinical Science Course, 2007–2008
Section 11

The American Academy of Ophthalmology is accredited by the Accreditation Council for Continuing Medical Education to provide continuing medical education for physicians.

The American Academy of Ophthalmology designates this educational activity for a maximum of 30 *AMA PRA Category 1 Credits*™. Physicians should only claim credit commensurate with the extent of their participation in the activity.

If you wish to claim continuing medical education credit for your study of this section, you may claim your credit online or fill in the required forms and mail or fax them to the Academy.

To use the forms:

1. Complete the study questions and mark your answers on the Section Completion Form.
2. Complete the Section Evaluation.
3. Fill in and sign the statement below.
4. Return this page and the required forms by mail or fax to the CME Registrar (see below).

To claim credit online:

1. Log on to the Academy website (www.aao.org/cme).
2. Select Review/Claim CME.
3. Follow the instructions.

Important: These completed forms or the online claim must be received at the Academy within 3 years of purchase.

I hereby certify that I have spent _____ (up to 30) hours of study on the curriculum of this section and that I have completed the Study Questions.

Signature: _____
                                                                    Date

Name: _____

Address: _____

City and State: _____ Zip: _____

Telephone: (_____) _____ Academy Member ID# _____
                  area code

Please return completed forms to: **Or you may fax them to:** 415-561-8575
American Academy of Ophthalmology
P.O. Box 7424
San Francisco, CA 94120-7424
Attn: CME Registrar, Customer Service

2007–2008
Section Completion Form

Basic and Clinical Science Course

Answer Sheet for Section 11

Question	Answer	Question	Answer
1	a b c d e f	18	a b c d
2	a b c d	19	a b c d
3	a b c d	20	a b c d e
4	a b c d	21	a b c d e
5	a b c d e	22	a b c d
6	a b c d	23	a b c d e
7	a b c d	24	a b c d e
8	a b c d	25	a b c d e
9	a b c d	26	a b c d e
10	a b c d e	27	a b c d e
11	a b c d	28	a b c d
12	a b c d	29	a b c d e
13	a b c d e	30	a b c d e
14	a b c d e	31	a b c d e
15	a b c d e	32	a b c d e
16	a b c d e	33	a b c d
17	a b c d e	34	a b c d e

Section 11 Evaluation

Please complete this CME questionnaire.

1. To what degree will you use knowledge from BCSC Section 11 in your practice?
   - ☐ Regularly
   - ☐ Sometimes
   - ☐ Rarely

2. Please review the stated objectives for BCSC Section 11. How effective was the material at meeting those objectives?
   - ☐ All objectives were met.
   - ☐ Most objectives were met.
   - ☐ Some objectives were met.
   - ☐ Few or no objectives were met.

3. To what degree is BCSC Section 11 likely to have a positive impact on health outcomes of your patients?
   - ☐ Extremely likely
   - ☐ Highly likely
   - ☐ Somewhat likely
   - ☐ Not at all likely

4. After you review the stated objectives for BCSC Section 11, please let us know of any additional knowledge, skills, or information useful to your practice that were acquired but were not included in the objectives. [Optional]

5. Was BCSC Section 11 free of commercial bias?
   - ☐ Yes
   - ☐ No

6. If you selected "No" in the previous question, please comment. [Optional]

7. Please tell us what might improve the applicability of BCSC to your practice. [Optional]

Study Questions

Although a concerted effort has been made to avoid ambiguity and redundancy in these questions, the authors recognize that differences of opinion may occur regarding the "best" answer. The discussions are provided to demonstrate the rationale used to derive the answer. They may also be helpful in confirming that your approach to the problem was correct or, if necessary, in fixing the principle in your memory. Where relevant, additional references are given.

1. The normal, aging human crystalline lens
    a. develops an increasingly curved shape, resulting in more refractive power
    b. develops an increasingly flatter shape, resulting in less refractive power
    c. undergoes an increase in index of refraction as a result of decreasing presence of insoluble protein particles
    d. undergoes a decrease in index of refraction as a result of decreasing presence of insoluble protein particles
    e. a and c are correct
    f. a and d are correct

2. Terminal differentiation is the process whereby
    a. lens epithelial cells elongate into lens fibers
    b. the mass of cellular proteins is decreased
    c. glycolysis assumes a lesser role in metabolism
    d. cell organelles increase their metabolic activity

3. When the ciliary muscle contracts
    a. the diameter of the muscle ring is reduced, thereby increasing tension on the zonular fibers, which allows the lens to become more spherical
    b. the diameter of the muscle ring is increased, thereby increasing tension on the zonular fibers, which allows the lens to become more spherical
    c. the diameter of the muscle ring is reduced, thereby relaxing tension on the zonular fibers, which allows the lens to become more spherical
    d. the diameter of the muscle ring is increased, thereby relaxing tension on the zonular fibers, which allows the lens to become more spherical

4. According to the pump-leak theory
    a. sodium ions are actively pumped into the lens
    b. only active transport is involved in ion movement into the lens
    c. sodium flows into the back of the lens along a concentration gradient
    d. ouabain can stimulate the pump cells

5. Which of the following systemic diseases is *not* associated with ectopia lentis?

   a. homocystinuria

   b. Ehlers-Danlos syndrome

   c. Marfan syndrome

   d. myotonic dystrophy

   e. sulfite oxidase deficiency

6. A lens coloboma

   a. is usually associated with previous lens trauma

   b. is typically located superiorly

   c. is typically associated with normal zonular attachments

   d. is often associated with cortical lens opacification

7. The epidemiology of cataracts suggests that

   a. they are more prevalent in those under 65 years of age

   b. they are more prevalent in women

   c. they occur only as a consequence of age

   d. they rarely lead to blindness

8. Risk factor(s) for nuclear opacification identified by epidemiologic studies include

   a. current smoking

   b. white race

   c. lower education

   d. all of the above

9. Which of the following statements about functional visual impairment caused by cataracts is *false?*

   a. "Second sight" is caused by lenticular myopia and improves near vision without correction.

   b. Monocular diplopia caused by cataract cannot be corrected by spectacles.

   c. Mild posterior subcapsular cataracts never cause visual symptoms.

   d. Cataract can cause greater impairment in contrast sensitivity than in Snellen acuity.

10. Which of the following statements about ectopia lentis in Marfan syndrome is *false?*

    a. It can cause monocular diplopia.

    b. The lens is usually subluxated in an inferior and nasal direction.

    c. Anterior dislocation is associated with pupillary-block glaucoma.

    d. Posterior dislocation into the vitreous cavity can occur.

    e. It occurs in a majority of patients with Marfan syndrome.

11. The risk of cataract development may be decreased by foods rich in

    a. vitamin A

    b. vitamin C

    c. beta carotene

    d. leutin

12. While performing cataract surgery by phacoemulsification on a patient with exfoliation syndrome, it is noted that the zonules are diffusely loose. If a small capsulorrhexis is performed, all of the following adverse situations may be accentuated *except:*

   a. anterior capsular phimosis with further zonular loosening

   b. increased resistance to nuclear rotation

   c. increased difficulty with nuclear chopping

   d. more rapid opacification of posterior capsule

13. The surgeon may estimate the patient's postoperative visual acuity potential with all but which of the following methods?

   a. pinhole visual acuity

   b. potential acuity meter (PAM)

   c. laser interferometry

   d. contrast sensitivity testing

   e. blue-light entoptoscopy

14. If a patient presents in your office with a mature cataract in one eye and a clear lens in the other, which test would *not* be helpful in deciding whether the patient should have cataract surgery?

   a. ultrasound

   b. blue-light entoptoscopy

   c. color vision testing

   d. laser interferometry

   e. two-point discrimination

15. What consideration would be *least* important in the decision to perform cataract surgery?

   a. difficulties with activities of daily living

   b. dense nuclear sclerosis

   c. withdrawal from interactions with others

   d. recent fall after entering a darkened restaurant

   e. failure to pass a vision test at the driver's license bureau

16. Which of the following questions is(are) important to answer prior to scheduling a patient for cataract surgery?

   a. Does the lens opacity correspond to the level of visual loss?

   b. Does the patient have a medical condition that would preclude surgery?

   c. Is the patient or a person responsible for the patient able to cooperate with the postoperative regimen and return for follow-up care?

   d. Will the patient's activities of daily living improve after successful surgery?

   e. all of the above

17. Medical indications for lens removal include all but one of the following:

    a. phacomorphic glaucoma

    b. phacogenic uveitis

    c. dislocation of the lens into the anterior chamber

    d. lens opacity obscuring significant diabetic retinopathy

    e. dislocation of the lens into the posterior chamber

18. Clear corneal incisions are associated with all of the following characteristics *except:*

    a. more susceptible to wound burn

    b. more difficult to construct

    c. less likely to be watertight

    d. less incidence of endophthalmitis

19. The goal of anterior vitrectomy is

    a. removal of vitreous from the wound

    b. removal of vitreous so that a posterior chamber lens can be placed

    c. prevention of CME

    d. removal of vitreous anterior to the posterior lens capsule

20. Topical anesthesia can include

    a. IV sedation

    b. intracameral lidocaine

    c. lidocaine jelly

    d. tetracaine drops

    e. all of the above

21. Which of the following preoperative measures has proven most effective in reducing the risk of endophthalmitis?

    a. administering oral amoxicillin beginning 3 days before surgery

    b. prescribing topical antibiotics for 2 weeks following surgery

    c. decreasing the duration of surgery

    d. administering topical 5% povidone-iodine solution at the time of surgery

    e. injecting vancomycin into the infusion/irrigating solution

22. During phacoemulsification, when the surgeon notes a tear in the posterior capsule, the first priority is

    a. finish phacoemulsification of the nucleus

    b. convert to extracapsular extraction

    c. freeze the action and assess

    d. perform a vitrectomy

23. Appropriate management of severe retrobulbar hemorrhage includes all of the following *except:*
    a. proceeding with surgery if the red reflex is maintained
    b. prompt and firm direct pressure on the globe
    c. observing the optic nerve and fundus with an indirect ophthalmoscope
    d. administering carbonic anhydrase inhibitors or mannitol intravenously to reduce intra-ocular pressure
    e. performing a lateral canthotomy if proptosis, increased intraocular pressure, and tight eyelids persist after other measures have been undertaken to relieve orbital swelling

24. If the posterior capsule ruptures and nuclear material falls back into the vitreous during phacoemulsification, the surgeon should
    a. immediately terminate the case
    b. send immediately for a vitreoretinal surgeon
    c. make every possible attempt to retrieve the lost piece of nucleus
    d. remove any remaining nuclear and cortical material from the posterior chamber and perform a vitrectomy
    e. never consider placement of an IOL in that case

25. All of the following reduce the risk of incision burns during phacoemulsification *except:*
    a. higher aspiration flow rates and vacuum levels
    b. viscoelastic aspiration prior to applying ultrasound and use of lower power
    c. occlusion of the phaco tip
    d. loose fit between the phaco handpiece and the cataract incision
    e. use of cohesive viscoelastics

26. All of the following may result in a shallow or flat anterior chamber in the postoperative period after cataract surgery *except:*
    a. wound leak
    b. pupillary block
    c. suprachoroidal effusion or hemorrhage
    d. posterior infusion syndrome
    e. ciliary block with aqueous misdirection

27. All of the following are risk factors for cystoid macular edema after cataract surgery *except:*
    a. diabetes mellitus
    b. flexible open-loop anterior chamber IOL implantation
    c. ruptured posterior capsule
    d. marked postoperative inflammation
    e. vitreous loss

28. If ciliary block glaucoma is suspected as causing a shallow anterior chamber after cataract surgery, all of the following maneuvers may be useful *except:*

    a. miotic drops such as pilocarpine to constrict the pupil, deepen the anterior chamber, and open up the trabecular meshwork

    b. aqueous suppressants such as beta blockers and carbonic anhydrase inhibitors to lower the intraocular pressure

    c. Nd:YAG laser disruption of the anterior hyaloid face

    d. mechanical vitrectomy to decompress the vitreous and disrupt the anterior hyaloid face

29. If the capsulorrhexis tear starts to extend too far peripherally, the following maneuver(s) may be used:

    a. Check for positive vitreous pressure and try to relieve any external pressure on the globe.

    b. Refill the anterior chamber with viscoelastic.

    c. Insert a second instrument through the paracentesis site to press posteriorly on the lens.

    d. Use the bent cystotome to try to redirect the tear centrally.

    e. all of the above

30. Evaluation of the cornea is important prior to cataract surgery. Which of the following statements is *true?*

    a. Corneal transplant surgery should be combined with cataract extraction when guttata are present in order to speed visual rehabilitation.

    b. Specular microscopy is the best means of determining how well the cornea will fare following cataract surgery.

    c. Normal corneal pachymetry measurements obtained in the early morning suggest that the cornea will probably remain clear following cataract surgery.

    d. Corneal pachymetry should be performed late in the day, after the cornea has had longer exposure to the environment.

    e. Other than determining lens implant power, keratometry does not have a role in the preoperative evaluation for cataract surgery.

31. Which of the following statements is *true* about the management of cataract associated with ocular trauma?

    a. After blunt or penetrating trauma in children, fibrin can be deposited on the anterior lens capsule that mimics the appearance of cataract.

    b. Cataracts associated with large corneal lacerations should be removed through the laceration to avoid making an additional corneoscleral wound.

    c. If a cataract does not develop in the injured eye within 10 days of the trauma, the patient is unlikely to develop a cataract later.

    d. Phacoemulsification through a small limbal incision is the best approach to the removal of any cataract associated with acute trauma.

    e. The benefits of inserting an IOL at the time of surgery outweigh the risks when removing a cataract during the repair of a paracentral corneal laceration.

32. A 3-year-old with a dense developmental cataract in the left eye demonstrates poor fixation OS and a left esotropia. The right eye appears normal. Which of the following statements is *true?*

    a. IOL implantation surgery should not be performed in children.

    b. The left esotropia should be repaired surgically prior to cataract surgery.

    c. Amblyopia therapy should begin prior to cataract surgery.

    d. Posterior capsulotomy should not be performed at the time of surgery because of the risk of retinal detachment.

    e. Cataract surgery with IOL implantation is a reasonable approach toward visual rehabilitation in this case.

33. A 50-year-old woman with myopia presents with complaints of monocular diplopia and difficulty driving at night. Her best-corrected visual acuity with a 2 D myopic shift is 20/30. On slit-lamp examination, she has minimal nuclear sclerosis. What additional examination is helpful to evaluate her symptoms?

    a. red reflex

    b. corneal topography

    c. fluorescein angiography

    d. MRI scan

34. A 76-year-old man complains of difficulty driving because of reduced vision. His best-corrected visual acuity is 20/70 OD and 20/40 OS. Goldmann visual fields are constricted, more in the OD than in the OS. A moderate nuclear cataract is present OD, and a mild one is seen OS. His IOP is 23 mm Hg OD and 18 mm Hg OS. He uses timolol 1/2% bid OD and dorzolamide tid OD. His cup–disc ratio is 0.8 OD and 0.6 OS. The fundus is otherwise normal. Which of the following statements is *true?*

    a. Cataract surgery should not be considered because of the risk of loss of fixation postoperatively.

    b. Cataract surgery combined with glaucoma filtering surgery is the only approach that should be considered for this patient.

    c. Medical glaucoma treatment should be maximized before considering cataract surgery.

    d. The visual field constriction in this case is probably caused by glaucoma.

    e. The use of latanoprost after cataract surgery may increase the risk of postoperative CME.

Answers

1. **a.** With aging, the human lens develops an increasingly curved shape, which results in more refractive power. This change may be accompanied by—and sometimes offset by—a decrease in the index of refraction of the lens resulting from an increase in water-insoluble proteins.

2. **a.** Terminal differentiation involves elongation of the lens epithelial cells into lens fibers. This change is associated with a tremendous increase in the mass of cellular proteins in each cell. The cells lose organelles, including nuclei, mitochondria, and ribosomes. The loss of cell organelles is optically advantageous, and the cells now become more dependent on glycolysis for energy production.

3. **c.** The ciliary muscle is a ring, but upon contraction it does not have the effect that one would intuitively expect of a sphincter. When it contracts, the diameter of the muscle ring is reduced, thereby relaxing tension on the zonular fibers, which allows the lens to become more spherical.

4. **c.** The combination of active transport and membrane permeability is referred to as the "pump-leak theory" of the lens. Potassium is actively transported into the anterior lens via the epithelium. It then diffuses out with the concentration gradient through the back of the lens, where there are no active transport mechanisms. Conversely, sodium flows in through the back of the lens with a concentration gradient and then is actively exchanged for potassium by the epithelium. Experimentally, ouabain can inhibit the sodium potassium pumps.

5. **d.** Myotonic dystrophy is not associated with ectopia lentis.

6. **d.** A lens coloboma is a wedge-shaped defect or indentation of the lens periphery that occurs as an isolated anomaly or is secondary to the lack of ciliary body or zonular development. Lens colobomas are typically located inferiorly and may be associated with colobomas of the uvea. Cortical lens opacification or thickening of the lens capsule may appear adjacent to the defect.

7. **b.** Cataracts increase in prevalence with increasing age and are a leading cause of blindness worldwide. They can occur as a congenital condition or as a result of trauma, metabolic diseases, or medications. Major epidemiologic studies confirm an increased prevalence in women.

8. **d.** Current smoking, white race, and lower education are all risk factors for nuclear opacification.

9. **c.** Posterior subcapsular cataracts (even mild ones) can lead to severe visual impairment, especially in bright illumination and when reading.

10. **b.** In Marfan syndrome the lens is usually subluxated in a superior and temporal location.

11. **d.** Physicians and patients are interested in lifestyles that decrease the risk of cataract development. Many studies have looked at nutritional effects with conflicting information regarding vitamins. Recent studies have shown a moderate decrease in the risk of cataract with the increased frequency of intake of food high in leutin (spinach, kale, and broccoli).

12. **d.** A small capsulorrhexis leaves more anterior capsule, which leads to greater resistance in nuclear rotation for quadrant removal techniques, as well as increased difficulty in chopping techniques. The zonular laxity allows the larger anterior capsule remaining to contract to a much smaller opening. YAG anterior capsular relaxing incisions can be made in the early postoperative period to reduce the anterior capsular phimosis, which can further reduce the zonular integrity.

13. **d.** Patients with cataracts may experience diminished contrast sensitivity, even when Snellen acuity is preserved. Thus, contrast sensitivity may be a very unreliable method for measuring visual potential. Although many patients find the blue-light entoscopy test difficult to comprehend, if they can see the shadows of white blood cells coursing through the perifoveal capillaries, macular function is probably intact.

14. **d.** With mature lenses, laser interferometry is incapable of passing through the lens to allow accurate responses. However, patients with mature lenses and normal macular function may be able to discriminate entoptic phenomena, color, and even the placement of 2 lights separated from one another.

15. **b.** The presence of dense nuclear sclerosis alone may not prevent the ophthalmologist, by means of a careful refraction, from improving acuity so that activities of daily living, interactions with others, stability in walking, and vision sufficient to drive (although perhaps in more limited circumstances) may be possible.

16. **e.** Each of these questions must bear on the decision to operate and be answered for each specific patient.

17. **e.** The lens may be dislocated into the posterior chamber without loss of visual function. Couching of the lens was an accepted method of restoring vision before lens removal was attempted first by Daviel in the 17th century. If the posterior dislocation of the lens is accompanied by inflammation or disruption of the lens capsule, removal may be indicated by a pars plana route.

18. **d.** Recent studies have shown a higher incidence of endophthalmitis with clear corneal incisions although the mechanism has not been demonstrated. (McDonnell PJ, Taban M, Sarayba M, et al. Dynamic morphology of clear corneal cataract incisions. *Ophthalmology.* 2003;110:2342–2348.) Both poorly constructed wounds and wound burns can lead to a leaky wound, which many suspect may be the cause of increased infection rates. Recent experimental studies have demonstrated that transient reduction in postoperative IOP may also result in poor wound apposition in clear corneal incisions, with potential for fluid flow across the cornea and into the anterior chamber, with the attendant risk for endophthalmitis.

19. **d.** Loss of vitreous is not a problem for the eye; vitreous traction is. When removing vitreous, the goal is to prevent any possibility of traction by removing sufficient vitreous to keep it away from other intraocular structures such as the IOL or away from the wound. Therefore, a vitrectomy is not complete until all vitreous is removed anterior to the posterior capsule, thus ensuring less risk of traction. This is the best way to decrease the chances of postoperative CME.

20. **e.** Topical anesthesia is a poorly defined term used in different ways by different surgeons. At its most basic, it implies no retrobulbar injection anesthetic. Topically applied anesthetics are often accompanied by IV agents, intracameral agents, or both. Each surgeon develops the combination of agents that best suits his or her surgical skills and the patient population.

21. **d.** Answers c and e are intraoperative measures, and admixing antibiotics into the infusion solution has not been proven effective in controlled studies. Oral antibiotics have a poor ocular penetration and are not recommended.

22. **c.** Early detection of capsular rupture is critical to the satisfactory resolution of this unexpected occurrence. As soon as the surgeon notes a rupture or suspects one, the first thing to do is stop working and freeze the action. This prevents further trauma to the capsule and allows for a calm assessment of the situation before proceeding any further. Without removing the phaco handpiece, viscoelastic can be instilled through the paracentesis port to freeze the action; the phaco is then removed. The next step is determined by the extent of the rupture, how much nucleus is left to be removed, and the presence or absence of vitreous.

23. **a.** If a severe retrobulbar hemorrhage occurs, surgery should be canceled, despite an adequate red reflex. All of the other measures are appropriate in the presence of severe retrobulbar hemorrhage compromising optic nerve and retinal blood supply.

24. **d.** Capsular rupture during phacoemulsification presents a risk of nuclear material falling posteriorly into the vitreous cavity. The case does not need to be immediately terminated. Attempts to retrieve the nuclear remnant from deep in the vitreous are not recommended, as that can result in more serious retinal complications. Nuclear and cortical material remaining in the posterior chamber should be removed, and a vitrectomy be performed via the anterior incision or pars plana. Conversion of a small rent into a posterior continuous curvilinear capsulorrhexis may stabilize the posterior capsular opening. Surgeons familiar with pars plana techniques may attempt a posterior levitation maneuver for larger nuclear fragments present in the anterior or midvitreous. An IOL of choice may be implanted with due consideration to the remaining capsular integrity. The patient may be referred to a vitreoretinal surgeon, who can wait up to 7–14 days to remove retained lenticular material without jeopardizing the outcome.

25. **c.** Occlusion of the phaco tip reduces or interrupts fluid evacuation through the phaco handpiece. This results in an increased buildup of heat within the handpiece and a transfer of thermal energy to the incision. Use of lower ultrasound power reduces heat buildup. Aspiration of viscoelastic, use of more easily aspirated cohesive viscoelastics, higher aspiration flow rates and vacuum levels, and a loose fit between the phaco handpiece and the incision all contribute to a more efficient fluid flow through the handpiece and/or the incision, reducing the transfer of thermal energy.

26. **d.** Posterior infusion syndrome causes shallowing of the anterior chamber during cataract surgery, not in the postoperative period. This rare complication typically occurs during hydrodissection, when fluid may be misdirected into the vitreous cavity, resulting in forward displacement of the lens. Wound leakage and suprachoroidal hemorrhage may result in a flat chamber during or following surgery. Suprachoroidal effusion, pupillary block, and ciliary block with aqueous misdirection occur in the postoperative period. Suprachoroidal effusion is often associated with hypotony and may be associated with a wound leak. Pupillary and ciliary block, as well as suprachoroidal hemorrhage, are often associated with normal or elevated IOP.

27. **b.** Flexible open-loop anterior chamber IOL implantation is not associated with an increased risk of cystoid macular edema (CME) in the absence of other risk factors. CME is almost always the result of increased permeability of perifoveal capillaries, typically induced by release of inflammatory mediators. Diabetes mellitus, rupture of the posterior capsule, postoperative inflammation, and vitreous loss during surgery are each associated with an increased risk of CME.

28. **a.** Management of ciliary block glaucoma is directed at controlling the IOP, shrinking the expanded vitreous volume, and ultimately reestablishing the normal balance of aqueous circulation. Medical management consists of cycloplegia and mydriasis with atropine 1% and phenylephrine 10% to create a larger anterior hyaloid surface area for perfusion of posteriorly sequestered aqueous. IOP control with aqueous suppressants like beta blockers, carbonic anhydrase inhibitors, and alpha agonists is very helpful. Miotics are expressly avoided, as they exacerbate the anterior displacement of the middle segment structures and may contribute to the initiating mechanism of the disease. If patients fail to respond to medical therapy, surgery is undertaken to reduce the expanded vitreous volume and disrupt the anterior hyaloid face with either the Nd:YAG laser or mechanical vitrectomy.

29. **e.** All of these maneuvers may be helpful in redirecting a capsulorrhexis tear that is extending too far peripherally. Preserving an intact continous-tear capsulorrhexis is very important to the ultimate success of phacoemulsification surgery.

30. **c.** Corneal thickness as measured by ultrasonic pachymetry is an important indicator of corneal endothelial function. Because the endothelium is under greatest stress after the eyelids have been closed during sleep, pachymetry should be performed in the early morning. Early morning pachymetry is a better predictor of postoperative endothelial function than is specular microscopy. Keratometry can be helpful in determining the quality of the anterior refractive surface—that is, the tear layer. If epithelial irregularity within the visual axis is not detected preoperatively, visual acuity after cataract surgery may be less than expected.

31. **a.** The surgeon must distinguish carefully between an actual cataract and an apparent lens opacity due to fibrin coating on the anterior lens capsule of an otherwise clear lens. Cataracts should never be extracted through a corneal laceration; this procedure would cause additional injury to an already traumatized corneal endothelium. Traumatic cataracts can develop long after the actual ocular injury. The use of phacoemulsification through a limbal incision would not be preferred when the view through the cornea is inadequate. In this situation, cataract surgery should either be postponed or, if necessary, combined with penetrating keratoplasty. When the lens is subluxated as a result of zonular dehiscence, a pars plana approach is preferred. Insertion of an IOL as part of a combined cataract extraction and corneal laceration repair procedure is controversial. Preoperative biometry is usually impossible and/or inaccurate, which can lead to significant anisometropia. Zonular status, as well as capsular integrity, may not be certain.

32. **e.** Lens implant surgery in a 3-year-old child with a monocular cataract is no longer considered controversial, assuming that the surgeon is familiar with the special techniques involved in performing such surgery in this age group. Strabismus surgery and amblyopia therapy should both be postponed until cataract surgery has cleared the visual axis. Posterior capsulotomy and anterior vitrectomy are usually performed at the time of surgery in a child this age. The posterior capsule usually opacifies in children and can become quite thick and fibrotic. Nd:YAG laser posterior capsulotomy is difficult to perform in this age group even if the capsule has not become fibrotic.

33. **a.** Patients with lens-induced myopia, symptoms of nighttime glare, and monocular diplopia often have a central nuclear sclerosis that, on slit-lamp examination, appears insignificant. Although the red reflex can be evaluated with the slit lamp, it is visualized more prominently with the retinoscope or the direct ophthalmoscope. When this finding is missed on initial evaluation, patients may unnecessarily undergo more expensive testing such as fluorescein angiography or MRI scan.

34. **e.** Latanoprost, a topical prostaglandin agent, can increase postoperative intraocular inflammation and result in CME. In this case, the visual field constriction is more likely to be the result of the cataract than of glaucoma. There is no mention of field loss approaching fixation, and with a cup–disc ratio of 0.8, fixation is not likely to be threatened by cataract surgery. Although combined glaucoma filtering and cataract surgery is a valid approach, it is not the *only* surgical approach in this case. Cataract surgery alone could be considered. Glaucoma filtering surgery could be performed as a subsequent procedure if needed. If combined surgery is performed, no additional glaucoma medications need to be added preoperatively. With an IOP of 23 mm Hg, cataract surgery alone can probably be done without additional medication. The surgeon must be prepared to treat a postoperative pressure spike if it occurs after surgery.

Index

(i = image; t = table)